D1452149

What You Need to Know about Asthma

What You Need to Know about Asthma

Evelyn B. Kelly

Inside Diseases and Disorders

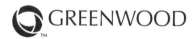

GREENWOOD

An Imprint of ABC-CLIO, LLC

Santa Barbara, California • Denver, Colorado

Library of Congress Cataloging-in-Publication Data

Names: Kelly, Evelyn B., author.
Title: What you need to know about asthma / Evelyn B. Kelly.
Description: Santa Barbara : Greenwood, an imprint of ABC-CLIO, [2022] |
   Series: Inside diseases and disorders | Includes bibliographical references and index.
Identifiers: LCCN 2021023285 (print) | LCCN 2021023286 (ebook) | ISBN
   9781440875571 (hardcover) | ISBN 9781440875588 (ebook)
Subjects: LCSH: Asthma. | Asthma—Treatment.
Classification: LCC RC591 .K443 2022 (print) | LCC RC591 (ebook) | DDC
   616.2/38—dc23
LC record available at https://lccn.loc.gov/2021023285
LC ebook record available at https://lccn.loc.gov/2021023286

ISBN: 978-1-4408-7557-1 (print)
          978-1-4408-7558-8 (ebook)

26 25 24 23 22   1 2 3 4 5

This book is also available as an eBook.

Greenwood
An Imprint of ABC-CLIO, LLC

ABC-CLIO, LLC
147 Castilian Drive
Santa Barbara, California 93117
www.abc-clio.com

This book is printed on acid-free paper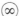

Manufactured in the United States of America

This book discusses treatments (including types of medication and mental health therapies), diagnostic tests for various symptoms and mental health disorders, and organizations. The authors have made every effort to present accurate and up-to-date information. However, the information in this book is not intended to recommend or endorse particular treatments or organizations, or substitute for the care or medical advice of a qualified health professional, or used to alter any medical therapy without a medical doctor's advice. Specific situations may require specific therapeutic approaches not included in this book. For those reasons, we recommend that readers follow the advice of the qualified health-care professionals directly involved in their care. Readers who suspect they may have specific medical problems should consult a physician about any suggestions made in this book.

Contents

CHAPTER 8
Prevention *91*

CHAPTER 9
Issues and Controversies *105*

CHAPTER 10
Current Research and Future Directions *119*

Case Studies 137

Glossary 147

Directory of Resources 155

Bibliography 159

Index 169

Series Foreword

Disease is as old as humanity itself, and it has been the leading cause of death and disability throughout history. From the Black Death in the Middle Ages to smallpox outbreaks among Native Americans to the modern-day epidemics of diabetes and heart disease, humans have lived with—and died from—all manner of ailments, whether caused by infectious agents, environmental and lifestyle factors, or genetic abnormalities. The field of medicine has been driven forward by our desire to combat and prevent disease and to improve the lives of those living with debilitating disorders. And while we have made great strides forward, particularly in the last 100 years, it is doubtful that mankind will ever be completely free of the burden of disease.

Greenwood's Inside Diseases and Disorders series examines some of the key diseases and disorders, both physical and psychological, affecting the world today. Some (such as diabetes, cardiovascular disease, and ADHD) have been selected because of their prominence within modern America. Others (such as Ebola, celiac disease, and autism) have been chosen because they are often discussed in the media and, in some cases, are controversial or the subject of scientific or cultural debate.

Because this series covers so many different diseases and disorders, we have striven to create uniformity across all books. To maximize clarity and consistency, each book in the series follows the same format. Each begins with a collection of 10 frequently asked questions about the disease or disorder, followed by clear, concise answers. Chapter 1 provides a general introduction to the disease or disorder, including statistical information such as prevalence rates and demographic trends. The history of the disease or disorder, including how our understanding of it has evolved over time, is addressed in chapter 2. Chapter 3 examines causes and risk factors, whether genetic, microbial, or environmental, while chapter 4 discusses signs and symptoms. Chapter 5 covers the issues of diagnosis (and misdiagnosis), treatment, and management (whether with drugs, medical procedures, or lifestyle changes). How such treatment, or the lack thereof, affects a patient's long-term prognosis, as well as the risk of complications, are the subject of chapter 6. Chapter 7 explores the disease or disorder's effects on the friends and family of a patient—a dimension often overlooked in discussions of physical and psychological ailments. Chapter 8 discusses prevention strategies, while chapter 9 explores key issues or controversies, whether medical or sociocultural. Finally, chapter 10 profiles cutting-edge research and speculates on how things might change in the next few decades.

Each volume also features five fictional case studies to illustrate different aspects of the book's subject matter, highlighting key concepts and themes that have been explored throughout the text. The reader will also find a glossary of terms and a collection of print and electronic resources for additional information and further study.

As a final caveat, please be aware that the information presented in these books is no substitute for consultation with a licensed health care professional. These books do not claim to provide medical advice or guidance.

Acknowledgments

I thank ABC-CLIO for allowing me to research and write about asthma. My husband, Charles Kelly, developed asthma as a young boy and had some flare-ups as an adult. Charles was always a great source of encouragement and support; he died while writing this book. I dedicate this book to his memory. I especially wish to acknowledge the support of my family—Sharlene, Kurt, Natalie, and Marsha—for their support during some difficult times.

I thank Maxine Taylor, senior acquisitions editor, for her guidance and patience through many projects and the ABC-CLIO staff for the many interesting projects. According to my count, I have written 10 books for Greenwood and ABC-CLIO, beginning with *The Skeletal System*. It has indeed been an adventure of learning and joy.

Introduction

I begin with a personal story. My husband, Charles, died at the age of 91. He had a long and happy life, but he did have one problem. As a boy, he developed asthma, and although the bouts with bronchial spasms later in life were not too severe, he had a constant fight with allergies, such as atopic dermatitis on the palm of his hands or hives when he mowed the grass. When the dermatologist asked him if he had asthma as a boy, he was puzzled. Why would the skin doctor ask about his childhood asthma? Yes, he had asthma, and his family traveled many miles to find help. He ended up taking "asthma shots" for two years, the treatment at the time. He had to sleep on a rubber mattress with a rubber pillow, and although he was an avid sportsman, he had to curtail his activities. Times have changed since the treatments of the 1940s.

Today, asthma affects 17 million people in the United States. It is the most common chronic childhood disease, and the incidences are rising in the United States and across the developed parts of the world. Costs relating to asthma are staggering. Treatment, medications, and lost productivity are over $11 billion each year. Asthma touches many people—if not directly, perhaps through family, friends, or colleagues.

This book has been written with you in mind. You may not want to read the book from cover to cover but rather choose items that are pertinent to you. However, I think you can find much value in each of the chapters.

The information in this book is provided for general background knowledge for students and lay leaders. It is not for medical advice or treatment. If you have questions, contact your doctor or health-care professional.

Essential Questions

1. WHAT IS ASTHMA?

Asthma is a respiratory condition marked by spasms in the lungs' bronchi; the airways narrow and swell, producing extra mucus.

2. HOW CAN YOU TELL IF YOU HAVE ASTHMA?

It can be hard to tell if someone has asthma, especially in children under age five. Having a doctor check how well your lungs work and for allergies can help you determine if you have asthma. A doctor will ask if you cough a lot (especially at night), have breathing problems, or experience chest tightness.

3. WHAT IS THE DIFFERENCE BETWEEN ALLERGY AND ASTHMA?

An allergen is a harmless substance capable of triggering a response that starts in the immune system and results in an allergic reaction. Asthma denotes a specific disease with specific actions of the lungs. The two are closely connected, but allergies are the overall cause of many conditions, and asthma is one of these conditions.

4. WHAT ARE THE SYMPTOMS OF AN ASTHMA ATTACK?

Bronchial spasms make breathing difficult and trigger coughing, wheezing, chest tightness, and shortness of breath. Some may consider the condition a minor nuisance, but for others, asthma can be a significant problem that interferes with daily activities or may even be life-threatening.

5. WHAT ARE THE CAUSES OF ASTHMA?

The number of environmental triggers of asthma is legion. Exposure to these factors can trigger or make asthma symptoms worse. The Agency for Toxic Substances and Disease Registry of the Centers for Disease Control and Prevention (CDC) organizes these triggers into indoor, outdoor, and occupational triggers.

6. IS GENETICS INVOLVED IN ASTHMA?

Asthma tends to run in families, indicating that there is a genetic component. It is not inherited in Mendelian fashion as a single gene but controlled by a complex of genes still under investigation.

7. WHAT ARE THE ENVIRONMENTAL CONDITIONS THAT MAY EVOKE ASTHMA?

Certain environmental conditions especially in the home may cause asthma. Smoking and being around smokers are the main culprits. Many home cleaning agents or chemicals used in home products can cause attacks.

8. HOW CAN ASTHMA BE MANAGED?

The management of asthma is suggested in steps, according to the severity or persistence of the disease. These steps include avoiding triggers and taking medication to counter acute asthma attacks.

9. CAN ASTHMA BE CURED?

Presently, there is no cure for asthma; however, it can be successfully managed. Current research proposes that likely, someday, there will be a cure.

10. WHAT RESEARCH IS BEING DONE ON ASTHMA?

Many scientists are involved in asthma research. Studies include basic research on genetic and biochemical causes to clinical studies of effective treatments. However, the bulk of future research focuses on personalized medicine, including identifying the relationship between type of asthma and specific biomarkers.

1

What Is Asthma?

"I was always told as a young girl that if you had asthma, there was no way I could run, jump, or do the things I was doing athletically," Jackie Joyner-Kersee revealed in an interview for *Medline Plus*. So, she tried to hide it from her coaches, afraid they would make her stop running. After all, she had received a prestigious scholarship to UCLA, and although she was a top student-athlete, it was at UCLA that she was diagnosed with asthma. She denied it for a while and did not want to believe the truth. Once she realized that it was a disease that she could control, she began to comply and do as her doctors recommended. In 1984 Joyner-Kersee won the Olympic silver medal in the seven-event heptathlon, and over the next few years, she won several Olympic medals. *Sports Illustrated* voted her The Greatest Female Athlete of the 20th Century.

What is this condition that Joyner-Kersee and others fear so much? What makes athletes ignore the diagnosis and refuse treatment? It is a condition that defies an exact definition. Even the symptoms may be hidden or denied, but eventually, the person will realize there is a problem. Another scary thought for the athletes is that doctors say there is no cure, but management is possible.

WHAT IS ASTHMA?

Asthma is a respiratory condition marked by spasms in the lungs' bronchi; the airways narrow and swell, producing extra mucus. This narrowing can make breathing difficult and trigger coughing, wheezing, chest tightness, and shortness of breath. Some may find the condition a minor nuisance, but for others, asthma can be a significant problem that interferes with daily activities or may even be life-threatening. Indeed, researchers now realize there are many different phenotypes and manifestations of asthma.

A LOOK AT THE RESPIRATORY SYSTEM

A major system is involved in respiration or breathing. This biological system enables the oxygen–carbon dioxide exchange to take place. Oxygen from the air is taken in and exchanged with the waste product from cells— carbon dioxide, which is then expelled through the nostrils. When you inhale, air passes through the mouth into the trachea, also called the windpipe; the trachea branches in the middle of the chest into two main bronchi, or branches. The bronchi continue to branch into smaller and smaller tubes called bronchioles. Around this network of bronchial tubes are layers of smooth involuntary muscles, which relax as you inhale and tighten as you exhale. You may hear the terms "bronchodilation," meaning the opening of the muscles, and "bronchoconstriction," meaning tightening to help you push air out of the lungs. These branches end with tiny balloon-like alveoli clusters in the lungs, where the oxygen–carbon dioxide exchange occurs. Air is pumped in and out by a strong muscular pump called the diaphragm.

As long as there are no obstructions, breathing is fine. But here is where asthma comes in.

WHAT HAPPENS TO BREATHING IN ASTHMA?

During an episode of asthma, several things occur. These events can happen separately or simultaneously. As described above, the pulmonary system consists of airways leading to the alveoli in the lungs, where the oxygen–carbon dioxide exchange occurs. In asthma, these airways become constricted. The lining of the airways have cells called mast cells. When an irritant such as pine pollen or cat dander triggers these mast cells, they release chemicals such as histamines and leukotrienes, which cause the smooth muscles to tighten, leading to airway constriction in response. The tightening causes the bronchial tubes to twitch or move, causing bronchospasm. The airways have tiny cilia, hairlike structures that aid in the normal clearing of fluids and other debris become congested. But the tightening can lead to the gathering of mucus that leads to more congestion and coughing. The inflammatory fluids cause the area to swell. If untreated or poorly managed, the airways can become permanently damaged; this is called airway remodeling.

These asthmatic responses can occur over days or within hours. Sometimes the symptoms may go away by themselves or with medications; they may worsen at other times.

THE ASTHMA-ALLERGY CONNECTION

In order to understand the pathology of asthma, one must understand the relationship between allergy and asthma. *Allergy* is based on a Greek term meaning "an abnormal response or overreaction." With an allergy, your body defenses are working overtime and become overwhelmed. The word "hypersensitivity" may be used to refer to allergies. Allergens cause allergies. An allergen is a harmless substance capable of triggering a response that starts in the immune system, which results in an allergic reaction. Many allergens can cause a wide variety of hypersensitive disorders. For example, one may have an allergy to pine pollen, a harmless substance, and develop coughing and sneezing every spring. Many substances can cause similar symptoms. However, asthma denotes a specific disease with specific actions of the lungs. The two are closely connected. But if you manage asthma and its symptoms, you must understand there is a difference between the two. Always remember that allergies are the overall cause of many conditions, and asthma is one of these conditions.

Note: Allergies and asthma are not contagious. You don't catch them or give them to someone else. Asthma is strictly an individual condition.

THE IMMUNE SYSTEM

This immune system is complex. It is designed to detect and oust foreign invaders. In allergic reactions, the system is working overtime and may be overwhelmed by the allergen. Allergic reactions are responses to various allergens, which one inhales, swallows, touches, or injects. The following is the process of an allergic reaction: allergen enters the body, and the person has an inherited disposition to this allergen; the person develops a type of antibody called immunoglobulin E (IgE), which is specifically targeted at sensitizing allergens. Millions of mast cells reside in tissues in the body; basophils reside in the bloodstream. Both of these types of cells have over 100,000 receptors that receive the IgE antibody. When an allergen (antigen) enters the immune system, the antigen binds to these IgE receptors on the cells' surface. When the allergic individual is reexposed to the same allergen that initiated the response, the IgE can bind to that allergen. When two IgE antibodies next to each other bind to the antigen, this interaction "wiggles" the membrane and causes the degranulation or breakdown of the mast cell or basophil. This breakdown causes the mast cell or basophil to release a series of chemicals that orchestrate the allergic reaction.

It's All in the Chemistry

When mast cells or basophils release these chemicals, the allergic reaction can occur relatively quickly. This part of the response is called the immediate reaction. However, some people also experience what is called a late-phase reaction. The tissues in which mast cells have released their chemicals may become hot, tender, red, and swollen for several hours.

The mast cells create this reaction by releasing chemicals called chemotactic factors, which then attract many other inflammatory cells to the site. These cells include eosinophils, neutrophils, and lymphocytes. Once they've arrived, all of these cells and the chemicals they release contribute to the late phase of the allergic response. The response develops as follows: eosinophils generate chemicals similar to those made by mast cells and release more generally toxic substances that irritate the body. Eosinophils play an essential part in late-phase reactions in people with asthma. Chest congestion can occur hours after exposure and can cause severe damage and scar tissue called remodeling. Later chapters will discuss the importance of treating this reaction. Neutrophils release several chemicals, including enzymes, which degrade proteins and cause further tissue damage. Histamine removed from the mast cells and basophils attract other inflammatory cells that cause tissue damage and constrict smooth muscles. Leukotrienes are potent chemical inflammatory substances, which is closely related to bronchoconstriction.

The immediate and late-phase reactions together combine to form a severe allergic response.

What Does This Mean for Asthma?

Asthma can have both an early and late response. There is a trigger (see chapter 3) that initiates the inflammatory response. The triggers stimulate mast cells on the airway and cause cross-linkage of the IgE on the surface. Immune cells have long memories. The cells then release histamine, which evokes the production of prostaglandins, leukotrienes, and other chemicals. At the same time, other immune cells called cytokines in the mast cell call out a host of other inflammatory cells and mediators to the lung, resulting in mucus secretion, bronchospasms, and wheezing. Bronchospasms are an early asthmatic response.

Next comes a later response, delayed by hours. Many inflammatory cells get into the act. T cells, a significant component of the immune system, come into play. These cells secrete multiple cytokines that intensify inflammation. Other cells, including mast cells and eosinophils, evoke the cellular response to inflammation and lead to the generation of leukotrienes.

Understanding the concept of early and late asthma has clinical importance in the treatment of asthma. Different therapies may be more effective at various points in the disease process.

SERIOUS CONSEQUENCES IF NOT TREATED: AIRWAY REMODELING

Perhaps the most severe asthma threat is airway remodeling, which occurs when the patient does not follow prescribed treatments. The lining of the tubes has epithelial cells, very much like the outside layer of the skin. Under the epithelial layer is a layer of mesenchymal cells. These two types of cells respond to the changes in the airway wall caused by prolonged exposure to inflammation. The base membrane, deposits of collagen, and smooth muscle enlarge, leading to thickening of the wall and affecting smooth muscle, which generates asthmatic systems. In terms of the immune system, asthma is a typical Th2 disease, as IgE and eosinophils inflame the airways. Biological agents with specific molecular targets for these Th2 cytokines are not fully understand and are being investigated.

ASTHMA FIGURES

Asthma has no cure and can be deadly; however, management is possible with proper caution and care. The condition is found worldwide, but the United States appears to be the primary center.

According to the Centers for Disease Control and Prevention (CDC), more Americans have asthma than ever before. For example, since 1980, asthma has been increasing in all age, sex, and racial groups. It is one of the country's most common and costly diseases. Some of the statistics are from data gathered in 2017 but reviewed for an update in 2019. The CDC has found that more than 25 million Americans have asthma, indicating that about 1 in 13 people has some form of asthma. It is the leading chronic disease in children. About 7.7% of adults and 8.4% of children have asthma. Asthma is more common in adult women than adult men; however, it is more common in boys than girls. Asthma accounts for 9.8 million doctor's office visits, 188,968 hospitalizations, and 1.8 million emergency department visits each year.

Deaths from asthma are many. Each day, 10 Americans die from asthma, and in 2017, 3,564 people died from asthma. Many of these deaths were avoidable with proper treatment and care. Adults are four times more likely to die from asthma than children. Women are more likely to die from asthma than men, and boys are more likely than girls.

Asthma disproportionately affects minority communities. African Americans are three times more likely to die from asthma. Racial/ethnic disparities in asthma frequency, illness, and death are connected to poverty, city air quality, indoor allergens, insufficient patient education, and inadequate health care. The rate of asthma and the prevalence of asthma episodes are highest among Puerto Ricans compared to all ethnic groups.

The Asthma and Allergy Foundation of America (AAFA) is a nonprofit organization dedicated to finding a cure for and controlling asthma, food allergies, nasal allergies, and other allergic diseases. AAFA's mission is also to educate the public about these diseases. One of its projects is to rank cities and asthma; it lists the losers and winners on its website. Out of the 100 cities, AAFA ranked the following cities the worst places to live with asthma: Greensboro, North Carolina; Birmingham, Alabama; Youngstown, Ohio; Cincinnati, Ohio; Louisville, Kentucky; Philadelphia, Pennsylvania; Dayton, Ohio; and Richmond, Virginia.

Published on October 19, 2008, *The 5 Best Cities for People with Asthma* include Abilene, Texas; San Jose, California; Seattle, Washington; Boise, Idaho; and San Francisco, California.

CHILDREN AND ASTHMA

Currently, about 6.2 million children under the age of 18 have asthma. In 2017, 1 in 12 children had asthma, making it the top reason for missed school days. However, episodes have declined in children from all races and ethnicities from 2001 through 2016. Emergency and urgent care center visits are highest among Black children under four years old.

ASTHMA THROUGHOUT THE WORLD

The World Health Organization (WHO) is a group that monitors and supports health throughout the world. Organized in April 1948, the group now has offices in more than 150 countries and is headquartered in Geneva, Switzerland. According to WHO estimates, over 235 million people have asthma, and worldwide, it is the most common disease among children. It is not just a problem for high-income countries; it occurs in all nations regardless of the development level. However, over 80% of deaths occur in low- to middle-income countries. Asthma kills around 1,000 people every day and affects as many as 339 million people—and its prevalence is rising.

The five countries with the highest prevalence of clinical asthma were Australia (21.5%), Sweden (20.2%), the United Kingdom (18.2%), the Netherlands (15.3%), and Brazil (13.0%). Finally, using the least stringent definition, the WHO estimated the global prevalence of wheezing at 8.6%.

Worldwide, there is an interesting phenomenon. Asthma is more common in developed than in developing countries. Thus, one sees lower rates in Africa, Asia, and Eastern Europe. In developed countries, it is more common among the lower class and economically disadvantaged, but it is more common among the affluent in developing countries. The reason is not well understood.

Although asthma is twice as common in boys as in girls, severe asthma occurs at equal rates. Women have a higher rate of asthma than men, and young people have a higher rate than older adults.

Beginning in the 1960s, global rates of asthma increased; however, since the 1990s, rates have reached a plateau in developing countries. According to WHO figures, the people affected are about 7% of the U.S. population and 5% in the United Kingdom. Canada, Australia, and New Zealand have rates of about 14% to 15%. Deaths from asthma in the United Kingdom were about 50% higher than the average for the European Union.

ECONOMIC BURDEN OF ASTHMA IN THE UNITED STATES

Asthma has placed a heavy economic burden on the United States. Economists Tursynbek and Krishnan (2019) published a study that included a comprehensive approach to estimating the current prevalence, medical costs, cost of absenteeism, missed work and school days, and mortality attributed to asthma. Furthermore, they studied the medical expenses of asthma with factors such as race/ethnicity, education, poverty, and insurance status. The study ran from 2008 to 2013 and included 213,994 people in the sample; 10,237 had "treated asthma," with a prevalence of 4.8%. The total cost of asthma amounted to $81.9 billion in 2013.

Total costs also included medical expenses and loss of work and school days. The researchers counted $3 billion in losses due to missed work and school days, $29 billion due to asthma-related mortality, and $50.3 billion in medical costs. The annual per-person incremental medical cost of asthma was $3,266 (in 2015 U.S. dollars). Among children ages 5 to 17, asthma is one of the top causes of missed school days. In 2013, children with asthma between the ages of 5 and 17 missed 13.8 million school days. That is an average of 2.6 days per child.

Medical costs are quite a burden. The proportion of persons covered by Medicaid was significantly higher in the asthma group (33%) than in the nonasthma group (17%). A smaller proportion of the asthma group (6%) was uninsured than in the nonasthma group (18%). Persons with asthma were also generally less educated and had lower incomes than their counterparts without asthma. On average, the total unadjusted medical cost of people with asthma was more than twice that of people without asthma; this was also true for the remaining five health-care expenditure categories. In 2012, the median annual medical cost of asthma treatment was $983 in the United States. This amount ranged from an average low of $833 in Arizona to an average high of $1,121 in Michigan. Children who were four years old or younger were less likely to have asthma, but the children in this age range with asthma were more likely to have asthma attacks (62.4%), emergency department or urgent care center visits (31.1%), and hospitalizations (10.4%) compared to children who were 12 to 17 years old. Medicaid was the most frequent primary payer among children and adults.

CONCLUSION

So what is asthma? In general, we can define it as a respiratory condition marked by spasms in the lungs' bronchi. Breathing is difficult, and coughing, wheezing, chest tightness, and shortness of breath may occur. For some, it is a minor nuisance; others may find it life-threatening. Asthma is a serious health, societal, and economic problem, not only in the United States but also throughout the world. This disease is multifaceted and has no specific definition. Understanding its relation to allergies is critical. Asthma is being studied extensively, and although there is no cure, it can be managed and controlled. Chapter 2 focuses on the history of asthma, an ancient disease, with many theories of the cause as well as many treatments.

2

The History of Asthma

Asthma has a long and fascinating history. This chapter considers the history of the development of the concept of asthma. We explore ideas from Egyptian, Chinese, Indian, and Greco-Roman cultures. We follow historical events through medieval and Arabic medicine, the Renaissance, and the 17th, 18th, and 19th centuries. The 20th century saw a significant increase in research with the development of tests for asthma and modern drug therapy. Chapter 10 continues with current research and future directions.

ASTHMA IN ANCIENT TIMES

The Greek writer Hesiod in *Works and Days* told the story that, at one time, the tribes of men lived on Earth free from ills, hard toil, and heavy sicknesses, which the Fates bring upon men. According to legend, when Prometheus stole fire from heaven, Zeus gave a woman, Pandora, as a gift to Prometheus's brother. Zeus also gave him a large box or jar with specific instructions not to open it. But Pandora was curious and secretly opened the box. When she did, sickness, death, and other evils flew out of the box. Only one thing remained, Hope, which had been caught under the rim of the jar and did not zoom out. But the rest of the plagues wandered among men, continuing by day and night to bring mischief to mortals. This story was the mythological origin of disease and death. Asthma was one of these diseases.

People in the ancient world knew about asthma. In Egypt, a great civilization arose with the pharaohs around the third millennium BCE, and their writings reflect concern for the health and treatment of people. The Egyptians also believed that humans were born healthy but were susceptible to disorders caused by demons and by intestinal putrefaction. The first Egyptian medical document is the Ebers papyrus, named after the archeologist who found it in Thebes in the 19th century. This document showed how Egyptians believed both earthly and supernatural forces endangered well-being. There were several books written on diseases and conditions and how to treat them. The Ebers papyrus mentions over 700 ways to get rid of problem breathing conditions. One condition, probably asthma, was treated by enemas (clysters), the administration of animal excreta (especially of crocodiles and camels), and herbs such as squill or henbane heated on a hot brick and inhaled.

The Chinese knew about asthma in the third millennium BCE. Chinese medicine was developed from older traditions and emerged in an exciting direction. The first textbook of medicine, *Huangdi Neijung*, represented the teachings of the Yellow Emperor, Huangdi (2698–2598 BCE). The Chinese proposed the idea of the life force, *Qi*, is classified as *yin* or *yang*. Diagnosing illness would identify excesses of *yin* or *yang*. The text tells of patients who were distressed, breathless, and made whistling sounds while breathing; the recommended remedy was breathing herbal fumes and extracts. Also, the text mentioned the plant ma huang, from which ephedrine is extracted and used for treating asthma even in modern times. The condition is not named in the text. Medical lore from China was later adopted by the Japanese and incorporated into their *Kampo* system of medicine.

By about 3000 BCE, a marvelous civilization developed in the Tigris-Euphrates Valley, known as Mesopotamia. Many of these kingdoms left about 30,000 clay tablets written in cuneiform that about the history and healing tradition. The main text, *The Treatise of Medical Diagnosis and Prognosis*, has some 3,000 entries on 40 tablets. It describes a list of ailments, such as the following: "The patient coughs continually. His breathing sounds like a flute. His hands are cold; his feet are warm." This description possibly could be describing asthma—although it did not have a name. The sixth king of Babylon, Hammurabi (1718–1686 BCE), wrote the Code of Hammurabi, which includes instructions for physicians. However, Mesopotamian medicine might be regarded as systematized sorcery, based on astrology, horoscopes, and soothsaying by examining the entrails of animals.

Precepts of Indian medicine, called Ayurvedic medicine, were written in the *Susruta Samahita* (450 CE) but practiced many years before. In 327 BCE, Alexander the Great extended his empire into India. His army was having problems with breathing conditions. He saw Indian practitioners using the smoke of stramonium to relieve such problems. Stramonium comes from a plant of the nightshade family and is commonly called jimsonweed. The drug is an anticholinergic, a type of medication that blocks the action of a neurotransmitter called acetylcholine from causing involuntary movements of the lungs. It also has many side effects. It is used in homeopathic medicine to treat children who have night terrors. It is interesting that Bram Stoker, the Irish writer who wrote *Dracula*, claimed stramonium caused him to dream about the horrors in his plot.

Greco-Roman Medicine

A young man growing up on the Greek island of Kos in the Mediterranean Sea knew that he would follow a great tradition of his family, known as the Asclepiads. According to legend, the members of this group were descendants of the god of healing, Asclepius. However, this school of thought developed a little differently from the traditional ideas of disease and healing that attributed illnesses to Pandora and the gods in Greece. Whereas many of his cohorts thought of medicine as theology or philosophy, the young man Hippocrates (460 BCE to 375 BCE) believed that health and disease resulted from natural causes, separate from the wrath of the gods.

Hippocrates lived in an interesting and prosperous era of Greek history, called the Golden Age of Pericles. Over 60 documents are associated with his name, including the famous Hippocratic Oath, which doctors take today. He developed a system of health called the four humors: yellow bile, black bile, blood, and phlegm. Sickness occurred when one of the humors was out of balance; healing involved restoring that balance. Hippocrates took medicine in a new direction and has the title "Father of Western Medicine."

The poet Homer used the term "asthma" in the *Iliad* in a nonmedical sense that described panting or distressed breathing. Hippocrates and his disciples differentiated degrees of breathing. He called moderate distress *dyspnea*; if it was more labored, it was *asthma*; if severe, *orthopnea*. Hippocrates described what happens when asthma occurs: A disequilibrium of the humors results in a flow of the evil humor phlegm, which arises in the brain, passes through the pituitary, moves to the base of the skull into the nasal cavities, and then descends into the lungs. This movement caused breathing difficulties and caused the person to gasp for air like a panting dog. His remedy was to encourage the flow of phlegm by vomiting, purging, and bleeding. Another strategy developed in the Asclepian temples included that of a special diet, hydrotherapy, massage, and relaxation with soothing herbs. Hippocrates was the first to connect these breathing issues to environmental causes, including climate conditions and location. He also related stress to an asthma attack and recommended that the person with asthma should guard against his anger. For Hippocrates, the breathing disorder was only a symptom. It was not until about 100 CE that another physician Aretaeus described the disorder. The name *asthma* given to the condition has stuck throughout the ages and is the topic of our book today.

Aretaeus (81–131 CE) lived in the first to second centuries CE in Cappadocia, an area that is now in Turkey and known for its mysterious caves. In his writings, published in 1836 as the *Extant Works of Aretaeus, the Cappadocian* (London Syndenham Society), he gave a good account of pneumonia, emphysema, diabetes, and tetanus. He also defined asthma and its development, listing cough, difficulty in breathing, tiredness, and heaviness in the chest. A wheeze during the waking state is terrible, but the evil gets much worse during sleep. The frequency of coughing increases as the condition worsens. He observed that although it may not be fatal, the parents and loved ones lived under a constant shadow. The remedy was drinking a concoction of owl's blood and wine, which, of course, is not an option today.

Roman medicine advanced some of the ideas of Greek physicians, with the superstar of the time—Claudius Galen (129–201 CE) of Pergamum—receiving lots of attention. Many of the physicians described a condition in which people gasped for air and could not breathe. They noted that if, from running or other work, breathing becomes difficult, it is called asthma. Pliny the Elder (23–79 CE), a Roman naturalist and writer, told of links between pollen and breathing difficulties and recommended the use of ephedra as a treatment for respiratory issues. Pliny, as a great student of plants, suggested a link between breathing difficulties and pollen from plants. He recommended the use of ephedra, a forerunner of ephedrine, an ingredient of red wine, as a remedy for asthma. However, he also suggested that drinking the blood of wild horses and eating 21 millipedes soaked in honey would help. Dioscorides, a Greek surgeon, serving in Nero's army, suggested the following for breathing complaints: dry and powder the lung of a fox, or roast a fresh lung, without touching iron in cooking, and then eat.

Asthma was known in the Hebrew culture. The Jewish Talmud (200–500 CE) consisted of two compilations of Jewish religious teachings and commentary that were transmitted orally for centuries before their collection by Jewish scholars in the land of Israel. The Talmud encouraged "drinking three weights of hiltith," a resin of the carrot family, as a therapy for asthma.

MEDIEVAL AND ARABIC MEDICINE

Rome declined and fell in the fifth century CE, heralding the Dark Ages. Medical ideas in the West remained at a standstill until the Renaissance. Avicenna (980–1037 CE), an Arab physician, maintained some of the

Hippocratic concepts but incorporated alchemy and astrology in his medical practice.

The great Jewish physician Moses Maimonides (1130–1204 CE) wrote his *Treatise on Asthma*, the first work composed explicitly on that subject. Maimonides was born in Cordova in Spain but because of persecution of Jews sought refuge in Egypt, where he became physician to the sultan Saladin. The sultan's son Almalik Alafdal was asthmatic and evoked the interest of Maimonides. He wrote the book in Arabic as advice to the young son. Later, it was translated into Hebrew and Latin. His advice was sound. He considered the dry air of Cairo to be preferable to the humid air of Alexandria and encouraged the young son to move. His *Treatise on Asthma* prescribed rest, good personal hygiene and environment, avoidance of opium, a small quantity of wine, and a special diet. Nuts, fruit, milk, certain vegetables, and legumes (peanuts are a member of this family) were forbidden, while "the soup of fat hens" was considered beneficial. He also discussed climate and its effect on asthma and the need for clean air.

THE RENAISSANCE COMES: 15TH AND 16TH CENTURIES

The Renaissance gave a new look to medical practice in Europe. Paracelsus (1493–1541), a Swiss physician and mover of the German Renaissance, burned the works of Galen and Avicenna as a symbolic gesture of breaking with the past. The discovery of the new lands of the Americas introduced new herbal remedies. In 1567 the Spanish physician Nicholas Monardes (1453–1588) wrote *Joyful News out of the Newfound World*, in which he described the dried root of the Brazilian shrub ipecacuanha to use as an expectorant. (An **expectorant** is something that helps loosen mucus so you can cough it up.) Sir Walter Raleigh introduced tobacco in 1559 for respiratory ailments. Soon, tobacco became a medical cure for just about any illness. Balsam from Peru is used this day in cough medicines. One historical case of asthma in the 16th century was that of John Hamilton (1535–1604) of Scotland, who was treated by the Italian Germano Cardano (1501–1576) of Pavia, who recommended he avoid feathers.

THE 17TH CENTURY

Many of the physicians of the day had asthma themselves. Jan B. van Helmont (1580–1644) was born in Brussels and was a disciple of Paracelsus. He suffered from asthma and described it as due to the drawing together of the bronchi. As an observer of some of the causes of asthma, he wrote *Oriatrike on Physic Refined*, in which he described a monk who is tearing down houses or temples and breathing the dust; he fell, like a Strangled Man. Van Helmont also compared an asthmatic attack to an epileptic seizure (the Falling Sickness) and deduced that it could be called "the Falling Sickness of the Lung." He is recognized as the father of pneumatic chemistry and invented the word "gas."

Thomas Sydenham (1624–1689), known as the English Hippocrates, treated a famous patient who had severe asthma, John Locke (1632–1708). Also a physician and philosopher, Locke was blighted by asthma, which often hindered him for long periods. Sydenham treated his famous patient with the same medicine as prescribed by Galen, as well as with bleeding and purging. Although a physician, Locke is known for his contributions to free and liberal thinking and especially his influence on the philosophy of the founders of the United States.

Other practitioners of the periods had quite bizarre treatments for asthma. One strategy was to use *drek-therapie* (animal excrement); especially prized was the dung of stallions. In 1618, the College of Physicians in their publication *The London Pharmacopoeia* encouraged using the lung of foxes, similar to the recommendation of Roman physicians 1,500 years earlier. Astrology was still popular. Nicholas Culpeper (1616–1664), an English physician and herbalist, maintained that "a physician without astrology is like a lamp without oil."

Two physicians, Conrad V. Schneider (1610–1680) in Germany and Richard Lower (1631–1691) in England, made an essential contribution to the knowledge of asthma. The two doctors from different countries challenged Greek concepts that were prevalent at the time. At the time, people thought seepage of fluid from the brain to the nose caused catarrh, an inflammation of the mucous membranes. Lower's book *De Catarrhis* (1672) was the first scholarly attempt using scientific experimentation to disprove the idea that nasal secretions are an overspill from the brain.

Two British physicians, Thomas Willis (1621–1675) and Sir John Floyer (1649–1734), added to the essential knowledge of asthma. Willis, a renowned Oxford physician, said that asthma breathing was severe, characterized by pursed or puckered lips. Breathing also involved a great deal of shaking of the breast. He divided the disease into two varieties: pneumonic and convulsive. He said that night attacks were due to the heat of the bed and advised sleeping in a chair. He prescribed antispasmodics, such as the spirit of hartshorn (made from the horn of a deer) and sedatives. However, if necessary, he would fall back on the powder of shells and millipedes. John Floyer (1649–1734), a British physician who himself had asthma, wrote the first monograph on asthma in English, *A Treatise of the Asthma*. He described the importance of how constriction affects exhaling. He also recognized that heredity, weather, seasons, occupation, infection, personality traits, exercise, and emotional passions all had an effect on the person with asthma. He tried many of the treatments of Galen and thought squill (Scillae), a small plant of the lily family, was the most beneficial.

THE 18TH CENTURY

This century saw some new and essential developments in the history of asthma. First, Bernardino Ramazzini (1633–1714), an Italian physician, studied occupations and how they may affect health. He is known as the "Father of Occupational Medicine." In his treatise, he described how handlers of old mattresses and dusty old clothes had bouts of asthma. These pieces were probably infested with the house dust mite, which has been connected currently with asthma. Another character of the Century was Thomas Dover (1660–1742), also known as Dr. Quicksilver because he advocated the use of mercury to treat various conditions. He developed Dover's Powder, which he gave to asthmatic patients. However, instead of helping, it tended to provoke asthma. Principle: **Certain medications intended to help may aggravate asthma; this is called an iatrogenic cause.**

Many of the great physicians of the century studied asthma. William Cullen (1710–1790), the great Scottish teacher, largely accepted the views of Willis and Floyer regarding asthma. In 1769, John Millar (1735–1801) wrote the treatise *Observations on the Asthma and on the Whooping Cough*. He was correct on the connection with whooping cough but confused asthma in children with croup.

Robert Bree (1759–1839), a Birmingham physician who suffered from a severe attack of asthma, produced an authoritative work on asthma, *A Practical Inquiry into Disordered Respiration, Distinguishing the Species of Convulsive Asthma, Their Causes, and Indications of Cure*. The work was so famous that it had five editions and was translated into five languages. In the last few years of his life, his asthma was so bad that he had to withdraw from medical practice. William Withering (1741–1799) found that foxglove (digitalis) was useful in treating certain conditions. However, in an essay written in 1786 called *The Spasmotic Asthmatic*, he did not claim that digitalis helped the situation but favored exercise, long sea voyages, and strong coffee.

THE 19TH CENTURY

Physicians of this century studied the anatomy of the pulmonary system, and their research contributed to the knowledge of the causes of asthma. In 1808 Franz D. Reisseisen (1773–1828) of Strasbourg showed that the bronchial wall had a distinct layer of muscle. When this layer contracted, it constricted the bronchial airways. R. T. H. Laennec (1781–1826), a French physician who was himself an asthmatic, invented the stethoscope. After studying Reisseisen's work on the bronchial muscles, he became convinced that bronchial spasm was an essential feature of asthma. His idea of bronchospasm was later confirmed by two researchers, Francois Longer (1811–1871) and Alfred Volkmann (1801–1877), who both demonstrated that the activity of the vagus nerve causes bronchoconstriction. Francis Ramadge (1793–1867) wrote several treatises when he was a physician to the Infirmary for Asthma, Consumption, and Other Diseases of the Chest. In his writings, he demonstrated an improved understanding of the physiology of the condition; however, his treatments were still using spa treatments and factitious airs.

Of the Victorian era, the most prominent authority of the time was Henry Hyde Salter (1823–1871). As a physician at the Charing Cross Hospital in London, he performed extensive studies on himself and his patients. His book *On Asthma: Its Pathology and Treatment* was published in 1860 and went through several editions in both England and the United States. The influence of the book extended well into the 20th century. He recognized that a person with asthma had spells and attacks but also intervals of normal respiration. He noted that some of his patients had reactions when in the presence of hay or animals. For example, one lady would not even pass by a shop where chickens were sold; she reacted in the presence of chicken feathers. Salter opposed the use of opioids and encouraged black coffee to relieve an attack. Another doctor-sufferer was the French physician Armand Trousseau (1801–1867), who considered asthma a nervous condition. Although he recognized his sensitivity to the dust of oats, he had a real attack when he saw a worker stealing from him. His treatment was a few puffs of tobacco smoke.

Sir William Osler (1849–1919) is one of the most influential physicians in medical history. He dominated asthma thought until well into the 20th century, and it was not until the latter half of that century that his ideas came into perspective. Osler considered asthma to be a psychoneurosis, and in his book, *The Principles and Practice of Medicine*, he said that all authors agree that in the majority of cases of bronchial asthma, there is a strong neurotic element. Therefore, he recommended the use of drugs for anxiety. It was not until 1968 that the psychic impact on asthma was objectively studied.

Several researchers implemented a new approach to the study of asthma. In 1853, Jean-Marie Charcot (1825–1893), known as the "Father of Neurology," along with Charles-Philippe Robin (1821–1885), a histologist, found unusual crystals in the blood of the sputum of asthmatics but did not make the connection with the disease. In 1871, Ernst von Leyden (1832–1910) noted similar crystals. These crystals were known as Charcot-Leyden crystals and thought to be the cause of asthma. In 1882, Heinrich Curschmann (1846–1910), in Hamburg, described spiral mucoid casts in the sputum of asthmatics and claimed these were the cause of asthma. In 1879, Paul Ehrlich (1854–1915) found eosinophils in the sputum of asthmatics, and this soon became an interesting focus of clinical pathology. Eosinophils are a type of disease-fighting white blood cell. Recently, there has been a connection between the asthma crystals and eosinophils, but the crystals and spirals are not of current diagnostic importance.

Role of Allergies

Astute physicians over the years had been observing that different people had different reactions to all kinds of substances. Several doctors throughout the centuries have advised patients to avoid feathers, smelling a rose, or even eating fish. John Bostick (1772–1846) was the first to give a clear description of the connection with seasonal hay fever and asthma. He suffered from the condition himself and described 28 other cases. Another John Elliotson (1791–1868), Professor of Medicine in London, gave a classic description of seasonal hay fever and suggested that pollen might be a cause along with contact with rabbits.

Toward the end of the 19th century, the importance of environmental influences was rising, leading asthma research in a new direction. In 1873, Charles Blackley (1820–1900), a doctor from Manchester, England, who himself had both asthma and hay fever, made an extract of pollen and scratched it on his skin; it produced a local reaction. He also applied it systematically to the nose, airways, and the conjunctiva of the eyes and produced the same results. In 1903, William Dunbar (1863–1922), an American physician in Hamburg, Germany, used a soluble extract of pollen to describe the same effect. It would not be until the early part of the next century that the term "allergy" became the preferred word.

Studying asthma during this century used reason and logic from observation rather than data. Tools were not available to the physicians for diagnosis. For example, John Hutchinson (1811–1861) devised a crude spirometer. The spirometer is a device used to measure the amount of air inhaled and exhaled. He developed this in 1846 not as a diagnostic tool for physicians but for the Brianna Life Company to evaluate candidates for life insurance. He also determined that pollution was related to poor health and found charcoal residues in the lungs of coal miners.

Drug Investigations in the 19th Century

This century also led to an interest in drug therapy for asthma. Several of the first plants came from Ayurvedic medicine and British doctors who were working in India. Dr. James Anderson (1738–1809), a naval surgeon working for the East India Company in Madras, was very interested in botany and herbal medicine. The plant *Datura feros*, also known as jimsonweed or the devil's snare, is a plant of the nightshade family. In India, people smoked the root of the plant, which worked as a relaxant for conditions such as epilepsy and asthma. Anderson, an asthmatic, confirmed the beneficial effect on himself and others and told an officer in the company, who later referred it to Dr. J. Marion Sims (1813–1883) of Edinburgh. Sims found it useful in asthma but substituted an English variety, *Datura stramonii*, or throne apple. Soon stramonium was on sale in the apothecaries as an antiasthma remedy. Henry Salter found the use of another plant of the nightshade family *Atropa belladonna* useful in the treatment of asthma.

People in Egypt and other areas inhaled smoke for asthma. When tobacco was introduced to Europe in the 16th century, some declared that smoking cured asthma. Many medications were combined with tobacco for use in cigarettes, cigars, and pipes. Brand-name examples included Grimaud's, which combined tobacco and cannabis, Cigarettes de Joy combining with arsenic, Marshall's combining with culebs, Crevoisiers combining with foxglove, Savory and Moore's combining with camphor, and then just plain stramonium cigarettes.

Several doctors, such as Floyer, Withering, Trousseau, and Salter, recommended coffee. In 1861 Adolph von Strecker (1822–1871) synthesized the active ingredient in coffee—trimethyl xanthine or caffeine. A close relative of caffeine dimethyl xanthine or theophylline was isolated from cocoa and synthesized by Albrecht Kossel (1853–1927) in 1895. These two drugs, in various ways, treated asthma. These researchers were forming the base for the development of pharmaceuticals through biochemistry, which would become an essential strategy in the 20th century.

THE 20TH CENTURY

From 1900 to 1999, researchers made great strides in both basic research and clinical medicine. A great revolution was taking place in thinking. Medicine was becoming not just observation, rationalizing, and gut feelings but requiring the scientific method of testing hypotheses, providing data, peer review, and other strategies. This chapter will end with the year 1960. The progress in both basic and clinical research, as well as the future of research, will be featured in chapters 3 through 10.

One of the great principles that gained notice was the importance of environmental influences and the pathogenesis of asthma. Blackley had collected pollen and systematically studied reactions. By 1906, researchers established the concepts of allergy, hypersensitivity, and anaphylaxis in animals. In 1910, Samuel Metzler (1851–1920) theorized that asthma in human and anaphylaxis in guinea pigs both involved the airways. His ideas provoked fresh thinking. The person becomes sensitized by inhaling, ingesting, or absorbing asthmatic material. This idea became accepted as fact, but finding the truth would occur in the following decades.

And then the dark clouds of war were gathering in Europe and the onset of World War I brought research to a standstill. America received the mantle for the continuing investigation. Isaac Chandler (1883–1950) of Peter Bent Brigham Hospital and Francis Rackermann (1887–1973) of Massachusetts General Hospital moved the sensitization idea forward. Rackermann was the second president of a newly formed group, the Society for the Study of Asthma and Allied Conditions. He also founded the Allergy Clinic. In this clinic, he found that not all patients responded to skin tests and divided them into two groups: extrinsic patients, who were protein sensitive and likely to react to environmental antigens, and intrinsic patients, who were protein insensitive. The latter group tended to be older and have more severe disease. These groupings had therapeutic implications and held sway for over 70 years when immunology became better understood.

Information about the pathology of asthma grew in this part of the century. Although relatively few people died from asthma, systematic studies of the causes were just beginning. Bronchoscopy has been performed since about 1914, but the results of biopsies were not reported until the 1980s. After World War II, doctors began to unravel the physiologic features of asthma. Many investigators made contributions to these advances. By 1960, asthma was shown to be related to transient increases in airway resistance, reduced forced expiratory volumes and flows, hyperinflation of the lungs and thorax, increases work in breathing, abnormalities in arterial blood gases, and right ventricular strain on the heart.

Names of pioneers of these works were M. Henry Williams (1924–2007) of New York, Solbert Permutt (1925–2012) of Baltimore, Jay Nadel (1929–) of San Francisco, and Ann Woolcock (1937–2001) of Sydney Australia.

MODERN OUTLOOK

To combat airway blockage and smooth muscle spasms, doctors prescribed bronchodilators to calm the asthma attacks. These medicines were dramatic and soothing on a short-term basis; however, they did not address the immune issues that cause inflammation. Over-reliance on these medications caused the number of asthma-related deaths to surge during the 1960s through the 1980s. Researchers began to address the causes of the condition and treatments.

In 1936, Edward Kendall extracted Compound E from the adrenal cortex and renamed it cortisone; the drug was later proven effective in clinical trials for rheumatoid arthritis. By 1940 it was shown that not just one cortical hormone but rather all steroids could treat it, and there were two categories of steroids: those that caused sodium and fluid retention and those that targeted inflammation. Doctors administered this drug to some people with asthma and found it useful. In 1954 prednisone and hydrocortisone were introduced as aerosols, and corticosteroids became standard treatment. Later, clinical trials showed the significant effects of corticosteroid medications in the daily management and control of asthma. By 1960 toxic effects that had been noted were described, and protocols to enable the specific use of lower dosages were recommended. Companion use of nonsteroidal anti-inflammatory drugs, such as phenylbutazole, began in the late 1950s. In the 1970s, methotrexate and other antimetabolites were introduced.

Methotrexate

Methotrexate appears to inhibit certain types of inflammation. It enables some reduction in corticosteroids while maintaining asthma control and spirometry. Coffee et al. (1994), in an important study, found that addition of this drug could reduce use of steroids in patients with severe asthma.

Albuterol

Beginning in the 1980s, albuterol sulfate became the rescue medication of choice for asthmatic worldwide. It was a great advancement in bronchodilator therapy for the time. The older bronchodilator Bronkosol had serious side effects and increased chances of sensitivities. Also, the earlier bronchodilators were of short duration; albuterol extended duration to six hours. At that time the first CFC-powered inhalants were used to deliver medications. Since, then these have been replaced by newer propellants.

The focus of treating asthma also has changed from just treating symptoms to long-term and anti-inflammatory therapies. Inhaled steroids, cromolyn sodium, and time-release theophylline were making headway in long-term management of asthma.

The role of the immune system in asthma has become apparent only in the last decade. Future treatments involve identifying and altering genes that cause changes in the lung tissue cells and how they communicate.

In 1991, the National, Heart, Lung, and Blood Institutes, National Asthma Education Program issued guidelines from an expert panel for the diagnosis and management of asthma. They emphasized how much new information emerged during the 1990s. However, they also highlighted many unresolved questions about the pathogenesis, understanding the trends of morbidity and mortality, and use of new therapeutics in long-term care. Many questions still remain. How do genetic factors, atopic status, and environmental factors interact to produce the symptoms of airway disease? Is asthma a single disorder with a unique cause, or a syndrome of multiple disorders? How does the cascade of inflammation work? What is the impact of long-term and anti-inflammatory therapy? These questions are being studied in research institutions across the nation.

CONCLUSION

Asthma has a long history of evolution, the study of which has led to the knowledge and treatments that we have in the modern world; however, it remains a complex incurable but treatable condition. It is impressive to note that ancient Egyptian, Chinese, Persian, and Jewish writers wrote of respiratory disorders. In the Middle Ages, the knowledge moved to Europe and physicians, and researchers advanced the knowledge of the effects of respiratory distress and had some unusual ways of dealing with it. The 19th century was a time of exploration and zeal to find answers to the puzzles of this disease. The world wars stopped some of the investigations in Europe, and the mantle for research became the responsibility of the United States. After these centuries of work by both known and forgotten researchers, the promise of respite for persons with asthma is developing. The emphasis on short-term solutions has given way to long-term solutions that solve the problems of inflammation. You will read more about the continued enhancement of asthma management, biochemistry, genetics, public awareness, and personalized therapy in successive chapters.

3

Causes and Risk Factors

Enumerating the causes and risk factors of asthma is a demanding exercise. This chapter focuses on many causes of asthma with discussions of indoor and outdoor pollution, occupational exposure, food and drug triggers, exercise-induced asthma, the role of eosinophils, and genetic factors. The "hygiene hypothesis," which states that people in the Western world may be causing infections by not allowing children to develop their immune systems, is introduced. Risk factors are related to the causes and involve people taking personal responsibility for their behavior.

ENVIRONMENTAL TRIGGERS OF ASTHMA

The number of environmental triggers of asthma is legion. Exposure to these factors can trigger and exacerbate or make asthma symptoms worse. The Agency for Toxic Substances and Disease Registry of the Center for Disease Control and Prevention (CDC) organizes these triggers as follows: indoor triggers of an acute asthma episode, outdoor triggers of a severe asthma episode, and impact of occupational experiences on adult asthma.

Indoor Air Pollution

One of the consequences of industrialized countries is that adults and children spend most of their time indoors breathing the air inside the house. Exposure to indoor air may have more of an effect on childhood asthma than outdoor pollens.

Biologic allergens are found in homes, schools, work, and recreational areas. The concentrations vary with particular geographic locations and conditions. Common among the biologics are dust mites, cockroaches, animal dander (which can be fur or feathers), and mold.

Dust Mites

Imagine sleeping or sitting on a chair or on a carpet surrounded by tiny things that you cannot see. It seems like something from science fiction. But in most of our homes, these creatures exist. What are they? Dust mites.

These tiny pests are microscopic and transparent. You cannot see them with the unaided eye. Hundreds of thousands of dust mites live in bedding, mattresses, upholstered furniture, carpets, and curtains. Their food is the skin cells that are sloughed off constantly from the body. These mites are not parasites, and they do not bite or burrow as other mites do. Their waste or fecal pellets and body fragments are harmful to some people.

For these people, the particles are potent allergens that cause breathing disturbances and asthma. According to the American Lung Association, roughly four out of five homes in the United States have detectable levels of dust mite allergens in at least one bed. But they can also occur in nearly all homes. Humidity is a driving factor for high concentrations of dust mites. They do not drink water but rather absorb it through their bodies; dust mites do not live in desert areas where humidity is low.

Dust mite allergens are a major indoor trigger for people with allergies and asthma. The allergens cause an immune response called allergic rhinitis, which can be mild or severe. The allergens are not airborne but cling to particles that are heavy and do not remain the air for long. That is why they exist in bedding and furniture. They can also live in cloth-covered objects like soft, plush toys.

The American Lung Association lists several suggestions from minimizing the effect of dust mites, especially for people who have severe allergies to them: reduce the humidity in the air by using air conditioning or dehumidifiers; remove upholstered type furniture or use furniture with smooth surfaces; eliminate drapes and curtains; cover mattresses and pillows to reduce mites; wash bedding in hot water at least once a week; remove carpeting if possible or use strong hepa-type vacuums to remove dust; dust with a cloth that will reduce the amount of dust stirred up in the air. Following these precautions does take effort but it does reduce the risk of exposure to dust mites.

Cockroaches

These creatures may not only disgust us as they scurry across the kitchen floor at night, but they can also trigger an allergic reaction. Particles from cockroaches, including feces, body parts, and saliva, can act as allergens when they are kicked up in the air. Cockroach droppings may be the most underappreciated allergens in the indoor environment. The National Pest Management Association reports that 63% of homes in the United States contain cockroach allergens; in urban areas, the number can rise to 78% to 98% of households.

The National Pest Association gives the following tips to help eliminate these pests from your home: keep the house clean, especially kitchen floors, sinks, counters, stoves, and the inside of cabinets; keep food containers and garbage cans sealed; fix leaks that would knowingly give roaches access to water; avoid piles of newspapers, laundry, magazines, or dirty dishes. If you see one roach, others are probably hiding. It is worth the investment to consult a pest control company or exterminator.

Cats

Cats and kittens are loving pets and lots of fun. However, according to a study by Wood et al. (1988), more than six million U.S. residents have allergies to cats, and up to 40% of atopic patients with skin allergies demonstrate skin test sensitivity.

Contrary to what most people think, it is not the hair or fur that causes the problem. People with cat allergies are allergic to proteins in the cat's saliva, urine, or dried flakes of skin or dander. Oversensitive immune systems can mistake cat dander for a dangerous invader and attack the outsider, resulting in such symptoms as coughing or wheezing hives; red, itchy eyes; and sneezing. Your allergist can run tests to see if you are allergic to these items from cats.

Although there are medical treatments, here are some tips to control cat allergies: do not hug, kiss, or touch cats or that cute little kitten; if you own a cat, clean the house often and vigorously; if you are going to a home where there are cats, ask to stay in the room without cats and take your allergy medicine two weeks before you go. Be aware that visitors who own cats can bring dander in on their clothes or luggage.

However, studies by Platts-Mills and others (2001) have shown that the presence of a cat in the house may decrease the risk of developing asthma. Several researchers have replicated this interesting and controversial position.

Other Animals

Furry animals and feathered friends may contribute to animal allergens in the house. It does appear that dogs are less uniformly allergenic than cats. Lindgren et al. (1988) did an extensive study of dog-specific species and found that dogs vary in the production of dander, which may be the allergen. There are some breeds of dogs that are hypoallergenic, meaning they produce less dander. Those who are sensitive may also produce allergy symptoms from contact with a substance in dog saliva, and also from dog albumin, a protein found in the blood. One can find a list of dogs that produce more dander on the Internet.

Some children may have pet white mice, guinea pigs, or other animals. These may present allergens. Birds and feathers may also be allergenic; however, according to the Institute of Medicine (IOM)'s major study called *Clearing the Air*, the real culprits may be dust mites associated with the feathers. These include feathers in pillows and clothes.

Fungi

People may be exposed to over 200 different types of fungi. Molds, the most common these in households, may lead to allergic sensitization and asthma. At least 60 species of molds are considered allergenic. These include the following: *Penicillium*, growing on bread and other foods; *Aspergillus*, black mold grows in areas where there is lots of moisture, like showers; *Cladosporium*, which forms olive-green to black or brown colonies and may affect health; *Alternaria*, found in carpets, wallpaper, textiles, window frames, and air conditioning systems. Exposure to these molds may cause nasal congestion, runny noses, conjunctivitis, sneezing, tearing, wheezing, chest tightness, and shortness of breath. According to a study by Etzel (2003), children are most sensitive to mold allergens.

Environmental Tobacco

Exposure to environmental tobacco smoke is a severe risk factor for people with asthma. Tobacco smoke from inhaling or from secondhand smoke is dangerous generally to one's health. The Environmental Protection Agency (EPA) has found over 4,000 different chemicals in tobacco smoke with more than 50 that are probable causes of cancer. Especially vulnerable are growing children and unborn babies.

Secondhand smoke is a mixture of the fumes from a smoldering cigarette and mainstream smoke exhaled by the smoker. Researchers have linked exposure to secondhand smoke to cancers, heart disease, sudden infant death syndrome, middle ear problems, and respiratory conditions.

Because of its toxicity to the lungs, people who smoke or who experience secondhand smoke have a higher risk for asthma attacks because their airways are overly sensitive. Just consider the following dangerous chemicals in secondhand smoke: formaldehyde (embalming fluid), cyanide (poison), arsenic (poison), carbon monoxide (car exhaust), methane (poison), benzene (toxin in cleaning solvent), nitro amines (cancer-causing compounds), cadmium (toxic metal), benzopyrene (cancer-causing substance found in gasoline and tar), aniline (poison used in dye), and polonium (radioactive materials). About 54,000 people die of secondhand smoke exposure each year in the United States.

Children with asthma and with parents who smoke have more frequent attacks of asthma with more severe symptoms. According to the Allergy and Asthma Foundation of America (AAFA), children whose parents smoke show less lung growth than children who do not breathe secondhand smoke; wheezing and coughing are more common. More than 40% of children who go to the emergency room for asthma live with smokers. There is clear evidence of an association between exposure to environmental tobacco and the development and exacerbations of asthma.

Environmental smoke is also responsible for more asthma episodes in teenagers. Fortunately, the number of teens who smoke has lessened in recent years, with only 13% of high school students saying they currently smoke.

Another item to be considered is thirdhand smoke. When one smokes a cigarette, chemicals stick to surface and dust for months after the smoke is gone. That is why you may smell smoke on the clothes of a person who smoked a cigarette hours before. The chemicals in the residue then react with other pollutants in the air, such as ozone. Because these have reacted with the pollutant ozone, tiny ultrafine particles less than 100 nanometers wide can make their way into a person's lungs, making them a more significant threat to people living with asthma. The particles also stick to the skin or clothes, where another person may absorb it through the skin or mouth. Mohammed Sleiman, a chemist at Lawrence Berkeley Laboratory in California, believes that these very fine particles carry and deposit harmful organic chemicals deep into the lungs. People who are very young and very old are especially at risk for these types of particles, which may be worse for those with asthma than nicotine.

Going into another room to smoke does not help, either. Airing out rooms or cars does not help. Open windows, fans, air filters, or confining smoking to specific places or outside does not reduce thirdhand smoke. The Surgeon General Report in 2006 stated that even separately enclosed, separately exhausted, negative-pressure smoking rooms cannot keep secondhand smoke from spilling into adjacent areas.

A new area of concern is that of electronic cigarettes (e-cigarettes) or vaping. Marketers of the devices say they are the safe new alternative to conventional cigarettes; however, as of August 2019, there are reports of one death and almost 200 reports of severe lung injuries of people using these devices. E-cigarettes are battery-operated devices shaped like cigarettes and are marketed as vape mods, Juuls, and vape pens. Because e-cigarettes heat a liquid instead of tobacco, it is considered smokeless and does not contain nicotine. However, they may have chemicals that are just as harmful. The CDC reports that vaping can cause lung damage and seizures after only a year. A preliminary study presented at the 2018 American Chemical Society meeting found that vaping could damage DNA. The relationship between these e-cigarettes and asthma has yet to be proven.

Combustion Devices

Combustion is a chemical process in which a substance reacts with oxygen to give off heat. Several devices may be used in the home to produce heat. However, if these devices are malfunctioning or improperly used, they can be a significant source of indoor pollutants that will affect asthma. Possible causes of these contaminants include gas ranges; improperly vented fireplaces; inefficient or malfunctioning furnaces; stoves burning wood, coal, or other biomass; and unvented or wrongly vented kerosene or gas space heaters.

This long list of indoor combustion devices produces particles into the air and gases that may exacerbate asthma. These gases include carbon monoxide (CO), nitrogen dioxide (NO_2), and sulfur dioxide (SO_2). And although CO is a significant health concern, it is not an irritating gas by itself but combined with the other gases and particles can bring on asthma symptoms.

Chemical Fumes

Chemical fumes in the home may come from surprising sources. The chemical formaldehyde, also known as embalming fluid, has a strong, pungent odor, and it can not only cause headaches but also bring on an asthma attack in susceptible people. Formaldehyde is in pressed wood products such as particle boards, plywood panels, fiberboard, carpets, drapery fabrics, resins, glues, cigarettes, and unvented and fuel-burning appliances.

Another source of chemical fumes is from household cleaning products. Even those labeled as green or natural may still have harmful ingredients, especially to people with asthma.

Some of these products release dangerous chemicals called volatile organic compounds (VOCs); others have harmful ammonia and bleach. Even those with natural fragrances such as citrus may be harmful. Many products also at risk include chlorine bleach, used to clean mold or other surfaces; detergent and dishwashing liquid; aerosol spray products, which may be for beauty, health, or cleaning; air fresheners; dry-cleaning chemicals; rug and upholstery cleaners; furniture and floor polish; and oven cleaners.

Mixing some products can produce dangerous gases. For example, never mix bleach or bleach-containing products with ammonia. For good health, be sure to read labels on cleaning and household products. The U.S. EPA does supply a list of products that meet its Safer Choice requirements for cleaning and other needs.

Other Inside Allergens

Products with latex may cause an allergic response either by direct contact or by inhaling latex particles. These symptoms can range from a skin rash to bronchospasms to anaphylaxis. Allergic reactions in the home may be triggered by latex in gloves, balloons, rubber bands, shoe soles, bandages, toys, paint, condoms, and various types of sporting equipment.

Pollen and Outdoor Air Pollution

For many years, researchers have linked asthma to pollen and air pollution; however, in recent decades, asthma-related cases have risen due to outdoor air pollution. Several sources of outdoor pollution include plants, industrial releases, ozone, traffic-related pollutants, and diesel exhaust.

Pollen from Outdoors

All kinds of pollens produced by plants on the outside may make their way indoors. For the pollens to be significant, particles larger than seven micrometers must deposit in the airways. Flowering plants are not the only culprits. Grasses and weeds produce pollen also. In Florida, sneezing from pollens is seen all year round, except in January. In the spring, pollen from pine trees coat cars and anything outdoors with a yellow powder; the fuzzy catkins of oak trees carry pollen that blows into houses or attaches to feet and clothes. However, according to the AAFA, the pollen capitals of America are Springfield, Massachusetts, New Haven, Connecticut, and Hartford, Connecticut.

Ragweed appears to be the most common cause of pollen asthma in the United States. This weed is common, especially in the eastern and Midwestern states, and one plant can produce up to one billion pollen grains. When the nights get longer in mid-August, ragweed flowers mature and release pollen. The pollen can travel in the air for many miles; it has been found 400 miles out to sea and two miles in the atmosphere. Seventeen types of ragweed grow in North America, including sage, Burweed marsh elder, and rabbit brush. Seventy-five percent of people who have allergies to pollen are also allergic to ragweed. If you have this allergy, you may also develop another allergy called oral allergy syndrome (OAS) when you eat these foods: bananas; melons such as cantaloupe, honeydew, or water-melon; cucumbers; white potatoes; and zucchini. This reaction occurs because your immune system confuses ragweed pollen with these foods.

Plants

Researchers have somewhat neglected this area of study, but specific exposure to outdoor plant allergens can exacerbate attacks. The organic dusts from several plants are especially important. The dust from the cas-tor bean, a plant that is prevalent in the southern United States, can cause significant issues; if eaten, it can be toxic, especially to children. The plant is from the same family as the poisonous gas ricin. The major allergen CB1A is very stable. Breathing the dust can bring on an asthma attack. Organic dust from soybeans may also cause asthma. A report in the *New England Journal of Medicine* accounts for a dramatic increase in patients sent to the emergency from the docks of Barcelona, Spain. Investigators determined that the workers who were unloading soybeans reacted to the inhalation of soybean dust. Dust from certain cereal grains can also cause asthma. Wheat appears to be the most common cereal involved, but others such as rye, barley, and rice may also play a role.

According to EPA studies, many asthma problems are associated with outdoor air pollution. Certain industrial gases, as well as odors from the products, are problematic. Shusterman (1992) found that just the scents of certain air products can exacerbate the symptoms of asthma in some people. Especially vulnerable are six million children in the United States.

Industrial release of the following has been found to cause problematic asthma. A prominent example includes aldehydes, used in tanning, pre-serving, embalming, and disinfecting. Aldehydes are used in fungicides and insecticides for plants and vegetables. Its most significant application is in the production of certain polymeric materials. A reaction between formaldehyde and phenol makes the plastic Bakelite.

Other Outdoor Pollutants

Heavy metals—cadmium, lead, and mercury—are common air pollut-ants and are emitted (predominantly into the air) as a result of various industrial activities. Uncombusted hydrocarbons come from petroleum, pesticides, or other toxic organic matter. Isocyanates are used for manufacturing polyurethane foam, elastomers, adhesives, paints, coatings, insecticides, and many other products. At present, they are regarded as one of the leading causes of occupational asthma.

Some communities experience hazardous air pollution as well as noxious odors. This type of pollution has led to the setting of National Ambient Air Quality Standards (NAAQS) for six pollutants:

- Ozone (O_3): some children with asthma have decreased lung function after exposure to ozone. In the United States, ozone causes a photochemical (absorption of energy in the form of light) reaction between certain nitrogen oxides, volatile organic chemicals (VOCs), and ultraviolet light.

- SO_2 (sulfur dioxide): irritates the upper airways; a bronchoconstriction response occurs within minutes of exposure.

- NO_2: both an indoor and outdoor effect.

- PM10 and PM 2.5 (particulate matter): a mixture of solid particles and liquid droplets often found in smog. It could also be in vehicle exhaust, forest fires, and atmospheric reaction between gases.

- Traffic-related pollutants and diesel exhaust. For those living near heavily traveled roadways, these pollutants may evoke wheezing and asthma, especially in children.

OCCUPATIONAL ASTHMA (OA) AND ITS CAUSES

This type of asthma is hyperresponsive to certain conditions in the workplace and not encountered outside the workplace. Mapp et al. (2005) found that occupational asthma is the most common occupational disease in industrial countries. The annual incidence implicates 9 to 15% of all cases of adult asthma. Four main types of OA are listed: (1) immunologic OA, characterized by a latency period before the onset of symptoms; (2) nonimmunologic OA, which occurs after single or multiple exposures to high concentrations of irritant materials; (3) work-aggravated asthma, which is preexisting or concurrent asthma exacerbated by workplace exposures; and (4) variant syndromes. Assessment of the work environment has improved, making it possible to measure concentrations of several high- and low-molecular-weight agents in the workplace.

According to Mapp, the identification of host factors, polymorphisms, and candidate genes associated with OA is in progress. It may improve our understanding of mechanisms involved in OA. A reliable diagnosis of OA should be confirmed by objective testing early after its onset. Removal of the worker from exposure to the causal agent and treatment with inhaled glucocorticoids leads to a better outcome. Finally, strategies for preventing OA should be implemented, and their cost-effectiveness should be examined.

The following workplace triggers are as follows: aldehydes, cleaning agents, detergent enzymes, diisocyanates, epoxy glue, hairdressing products, latex, platinum salts, and wood dust.

According to the CDC, workplace allergies are more common than one might think. An estimated 1.9 million cases of asthma among adults were work-related, accounting for 15.7% of current adult asthma cases. Work-related asthma significantly differs by age and is highest among persons aged 45 to 64 years (20.7%). Asthma prevalence was highest among workers in the health-care and social assistance industries, with 8.8% of workers reporting that they had asthma at the time of the survey. Participants in the educational services industry reported the second-highest rate of asthma at 8.2%. Among workers in the wood products manufacturing industry, 57.3% reported having an asthma attack in the past year, which was the highest rate of all industries. Workers in the plastics and rubber products manufacturing were second most likely to suffer from an asthma attack, at a rate of 56.7%.

FOOD AND DRUG TRIGGERS

One seldom has an asthma attack from foods, but if a person is allergic to a specific food, he or she may have symptoms that mimic asthma. It is very important, if you suspect you are allergic to a certain food, to have a procedure in which the doctor performs skin tests to find out if you are sensitive to certain foods. The following is a list of foods that an individual may be allergic to and that may evoke asthma-like symptoms: peanuts and tree nuts, eggs, cow's milk, soy products, wheat, fish, shrimp, and shellfish.

Certain food preservatives and additives can also trigger an attack. Especially implicated are sodium bisulfite, potassium bisulfite, sodium metabisulfite, potassium metabisulfite, and sodium sulfite. These chemicals are commonly used in processing dried fruits and vegetables; packaged and prepared potatoes; wine and beer; fresh, frozen, or cooked shrimp; and pickled foods.

Adverse allergies to drugs are also quite rare. Drug allergies are a reaction of the immune system to a normally harmless substance. Some people with asthma have sensitivities to certain medications that can precipitate an attack. Some medications, both prescription and over-the-counter, are trigger symptoms. Aspirin and other painkillers are known suspects. About 20% of adults with asthma are sensitive to nonsteroidal anti-inflammatory drugs (NSAIDs), such as ibuprofen (Motrin, Advil) and naproxen (Aleve, Naprosyn). Products with acetaminophen or Tylenol are considered safe;

however, some studies have also linked this drug to asthma conditions. Two commonly prescribed medications, such as beta-blockers, which doctors prescribe for heart conditions, high blood pressure, migraine, and glaucoma, and angiotensin-converting enzyme (ACE) inhibitors used to treat heart disease and high blood pressure, may also trigger symptoms. If a person using these drugs develops a cough and asthma-like symptoms, he or she should confer with a physician.

EXERCISE-INDUCED BRONCHOSPASMS

At one time, it was called exercise-induced asthma; now, the name is exercise-induced bronchoconstriction, or EIB. These symptoms occur when airways narrow as a result of physical activity, which may be track, swimming, tennis, or any just heavy exercise. If one has asthma, there is a 90% chance that he or she will develop EIB; however, with exercise, one may have bronchoconstriction and not have asthma. Many world-class athletes have EIB, including several Olympic medal winners. For those who are interested in these activities, the prospects of EIB should not inhibit you. The important thing is knowing what to do to manage it.

There are reasons that EIB develops. When breathing in air that is drier than the air in the body, the airways lose water and heat. For years, people thought that cold air caused the difficulties, but current studies indicate that dry air, rather than temperature, is more likely the trigger. Cold air may be drier, and breathing in quickly dehydrates the bronchial tubes, causing the constriction.

Many of the "cold-weather sports," such as ice hockey, ice skating, cross-country skiing, as well as activities like soccer, basketball, and long-distance running, may evoke the symptoms of asthma. Those that are least likely to trigger symptoms include walking, hiking, biking, or other sports that require only short bursts of activity. Also, volleyball, gymnastics, wrestling, golf, swimming, football, and short-distance track and field games require shorter bursts of energy. Interestingly, swimming may demand constant activity, but the warmth and humidity of the water make it easier for people to breathe.

The following are common symptoms of EIB: tightness in the chest, shortness of breath or wheezing, cough, decreased endurance, upset stomach, and sore throat. The symptoms may appear within a few minutes and continue for 10 to 15 minutes after the person stops the activity. However, if someone is out of shape or has no training, he or she may experience more severe EIB symptoms.

Other triggers may relate to specific sports. Examples are heavy chlorine in pools when swimming, running or cycling in polluted areas, cold dry air in ice areas for hockey or ice skating, the gym may have new paint, equipment or carpet, or someone in the audience may have heavy perfume.

Almost every athlete at some time in the career has difficulty breathing, and avoiding EIB is essential. The following suggestions may help lower the risk for EIB: practice warm-up and event exercises for about 15 minutes before beginning the more strenuous activity; in cold weather, cover your mouth and nose with a scarf or face mask; breathing through the nose when exercising will help warm the air that goes to the lungs; avoid triggers; if necessary, see an allergist for prescription medication; these may be more effective than over-the-counter medicines.

ROLE OF EOSINOPHILS

At one time, doctors thought of asthma as just one disease, but current research has shown there are several types. One of the most severe kinds is called eosinophilic asthma (EA), which occurs when the person has high levels of a type of white blood cell called an eosinophil. Eosinophils are a natural part of the immune system.

This rare subtype of asthma means frequent severe asthma attacks and is found more frequently in adults, although children may have it. Some new biological medications target this particular type of asthma. See chapter 10, "Current Research and Future Directions."

GENETIC RISK FACTORS

Although not everyone in the family will have asthma, it does tend to run in families. Someone in the family may have allergies to food or drugs, or atopic dermatitis. These allergies, although not explicitly related, are part of a large family, of which asthma may manifest itself.

The search is on for the genes associated with asthma. People may inherit one or more of associated genes and not have the condition itself. Asthma is a very complex combination of genes and the environment. In other words, genetics may load the gun, but environment pulls the trigger. Many essential risk factors involve allergies, respiratory infections, and exposure to secondhand smoke. It is essential to know your family history.

Chapter 10, "Current Research and Future Directions," will feature a segment of the research on the genetics of asthma. It will also include new drugs for this condition and associated allergies.

FETAL AND INFANT ORIGINS OF ASTHMA

With asthma so prevalent in many countries worldwide, researchers have determined the importance of the relationship between fetal life and infancy with asthma. Several epidemiological studies have suggested that asthma, like other common diseases, originates in early life. Long-term follow-up studies have found that impaired respiratory health and lung function in early childhood is associated with respiratory ailments in later life.

Duijts (2012) reviewed related studies and found that the origins of childhood asthma are associated with a low birth weight, chronic obstructive airway disease, and impaired lung function in adults. The developmental plasticity hypothesis suggests that response to various adverse adaptations in fetal life and early childhood is associated with low birth weight and diseases in later life. These adaptations might result in impaired lung growth, leading to smaller airways, decreased lung volume, and increased risk of asthma or chronic obstructive pulmonary disease (COPD) throughout postnatal life. Other adaptive mechanisms include an innate or skewed helper T immune system, increase sensitivity to allergens, and inflammation.

Maternal smoking is the most critical adverse fetal exposure in Western countries and is strongly associated with fetal growth retardation and low birth weight. Studies have shown that maternal smoking during pregnancy is associated with increased risks of wheezing and asthma during childhood. The mechanisms are not entirely understood, but recent studies indicated changes in general and biological pathways different in DNA methylation and specific genes that alter growth and lung development.

Suboptimal fetal nutrition due to maternal underweight, obesity, insufficient dietary intake, or placental dysfunction might also affect fetal growth and lung development. Lower intake of micronutrients, such as folate and vitamin B12, appear to influence epigenetic mechanisms in the mother's diet, causing a higher incidence of asthma and wheezing.

After birth, the infant's diet may also influence body and lung growth development. The introduction of bottle feeding or solid food, instead of breastfeeding, may reduce lung and airway growth and childhood asthma.

Childhood asthma is related to respiratory tract infections. Organisms such as *S. aureus* are associated with a risk of atopic dermatitis and other allergies. Acetaminophen, given to reduce fever in children, including those with upper and lower respiratory tract infections, is associated with the risk of childhood asthma. Acetaminophen appears to deplete airway mucosal glutathione and could contribute to lung stress.

WEATHER

Although the weather is not a symptom, it is undoubtedly related to the worsening of symptoms; it can be cold weather, hot weather, stormy weather, or humid weather.

Cold Weather

Let us look first at very cold weather, with snow on the ground and wind blowing. Or the weather can be cold, foggy, and damp. The person then notices that asthma symptoms worsen. There are several reasons for this. Cold weather in the airways can trigger a spasm, causing coughing, wheezing, shortness of breath, and chest tightness. Pollution is worse on cold days when more cold and flu viruses are around.

If one exercises in cold air, they will not warm their breath before it reaches the lungs. Because the body keeps the interior organs at a consistently warm temperature, cold air can shock the lungs. This condition makes the person breathe rapidly; the lungs become inflamed, leading to an asthma attack. Cold air is usually arid, which can irritate even healthy lungs. Because people with asthma already have weak lungs, the dry air affects them even more severely and brings on an attack.

Hot Weather

Although most of us think of cold weather as being the main culprit for asthma, hot summer weather can also bring on the symptoms. When one breathes hot, stifling air, airways narrow, leading to coughing and shortness of breath. The hot, humid air of summer may also bring a higher level of pollutants, allergens like dust mites, molds, and ozone.

Thunderstorm Asthma

A hard rain from a thunderstorm hits pollen grains, making them smaller and more comfortable to inhale. The winds carry pollen to many places. An unusual occurrence happened in Melbourne, Australia, in November 2016. Bombarding rain from a severe thunderstorm affected the pollen grains of many blooming plants, causing the pollen to absorb moisture, burst into fragments, and then be blown by the winds. These smaller pollen grains were able to bypass the cleansing mechanisms in the nose and enter the lungs, triggering a large number of asthma attacks. The outbreak overwhelmed the ambulance system and local hospitals. Although many of the people had no previous asthma symptoms, nine deaths occurred as a result of "thunderstorm asthma." Most affected people had a history of hay fever, and 96% tested positive for grass pollen allergies, especially ryegrass. Ryegrass can hold up to 700 tiny starch particles that are small enough to reach the lungs' lower airways.

The phenomenon of thunderstorm asthma was first recognized in this event in Melbourne in 2016. Since then, there have been other widespread asthma attacks in Wagga Wagga, Australia; London, England; Naples, Italy; and Atlanta, in the United States.

THE HYGIENE HYPOTHESIS

Can our obsession with cleanliness be causing diseases and disorders in the lives of children? In 1968, some researchers linked the idea between parasites and immune disorders. In 1989, the theory challenged the thought of health and hygiene that was prevalent in the Western world. It was called the "Hygiene Hypothesis." David Strachan, in Great Britain, proposed that a lower incidence of infection in early childhood could be the explanation for the rise in allergic diseases, such as asthma and hay fever. This hypothesis suggested that during the critical postnatal period of development, household chemicals derail the immune system. The young child's environment may be too clean to pose a practical challenge to a mature immune system.

Epidemiologic studies showing that allergic diseases and asthma occur when the incidence of endotoxin or bacterial lipopolysaccharide (LPS) in the bloodstream is low support this theory. LPS is a bacterial molecule that educates the immune system by triggering appropriate switches.

Other researchers dispute this hypothesis and claim it is damaging to public health. A discussion of the science behind the rationale for the hygiene hypothesis and the 2019 challenge to the idea is fully explored in chapter 9, "Issues and Controversies."

CONCLUSION

The causes and risk factors of asthma are legion. The environment that a person lives in is critical to developing good health. People with asthma have many challenges from pollution. In industrialized countries, people spend most of their time indoors, and the indoor pollutants from biologic allergens such as dust mites, mold, and cockroach bits exacerbate asthma.

Another problem is firsthand, secondhand, and even thirdhand smoke. Smoke particles can adhere to furniture or clothing and cause an attack. Outdoor air pollution is more common in some communities but can be found in almost every area, especially if there are factory emissions. Occupational asthma may also affect people who have specific jobs—so much that they may have to change jobs.

Genetics may well play a role in the development of asthma, and specific genes combined with a risk-filled environment may develop into severe attacks.

Knowing risk factors is essential to being aware of what to do and what to avoid. Personal responsibility is important here. Knowledge about the disease and its risk factors are crucial. Likewise, knowing when to get medical attention from an allergist is critical. Chapter 4 will address the complex signs and symptoms of asthma.

4

Signs and Symptoms

Asthma is a common long-term inflammatory disease of the airways of the lungs. The signs and symptoms of asthma are many. Some people may experience many symptoms; others may have only a few of the symptoms. This chapter discusses wheezing, shortness of breath, coughing, chest tightness and pain, nocturnal asthma, and effects of weather—including cold air, hot air, and thunderstorm asthma. Dangerous symptoms, such as fainting, cyanosis (turning blue), fatigue, cognitive impairment, disorientation, and any of the sudden or extreme signs, are also discussed. The discussions will consist of the physiology and mechanisms of each of the symptoms.

WHEEZING

In Egypt, they described having major respiratory problems as sounding like a person was blowing through a reed. This is an appropriate way to describe wheezing. When the person breathes, he or she makes a high-pitched, coarse, whistling sound. Wheezing is a primary symptom of respiratory disorder asthma. However, it may also be present in acute bronchitis, heart failure, COPD, emphysema, or severe allergies.

In asthma, the airways are closed due to inflammation, mucus, and airway muscle spasms. The small airways of the lungs become narrow or constricted. Although it is one symptom of asthma, people need to be aware that asthma is not the only cause of wheezing.

Studies in babies and children have found several types of wheezing in young children. Types of wheezing include temporary wheezing or transient wheezing, persistent wheezing, and bronchiolitis.

Wheezing is expected in the first few years of life when the airways are relatively small. This wheezing does not mean the child has asthma, although it may be frightening to parents. Transient wheezing occurs in more than half of all children. Wheezing usually occurs when the child has an infection, stops gradually, and then goes away when the infection clears. This type of wheezing usually stops altogether by about three years of age, when airways grow and widen.

Persistent wheezing occurs in children when wheezing continues beyond the preschool years. Some children may have other allergic conditions, such as eczema, hay fever, or other allergic conditions, without a cold. It can be difficult to tell whether a child has transient or persistent wheezing.

Bronchiolitis is an actual illness. Commonly caused by viruses, bronchiolitis can result in transient wheezing in babies and children under the age of 12. If a child has bronchiolitis, it does not mean that he or she will develop asthma, and when the child gets better, this type of wheezing may disappear.

The Science of Wheezing

Wheezing's whistling sound results from the narrowing of the airways or obstruction of the larynx to the small bronchi. Several things may cause airway narrowing, officially called bronchoconstriction. Swelling of the mucosal linings; external compressions; or partial obstruction by a tumor, foreign body, or many secretions can occur. Vibrations or oscillations of the partially closed airway walls generate wheezing. Air passes through this narrowed portion of an airway at high speed, producing decreased gas and flows in the constricted region. This occurrence reflects a principle demonstrated by the Swiss scientist Daniel Bernoulli (1700–1782), which states that pressure in a liquid or gas decreases as the liquid or gas moves faster. According to Bernoulli's principle, the internal airway pressure begins to increase and barely reopens the airway lumen, the bronchi's inside space. Alternation of the airways occurs between the nearly closed and nearly open condition and produces a fluttering of the airway walls that results in the musical "continuous" sound. The airflow rate determines the pitch, intensity, and tone of the notes. The sound can be one sound (monophonic), or many different sounds (polyphonic). The timing appears long or short, depending on whether air is being inhaled or exhaled.

During expiration, the airways usually narrow, and wheezing is more common during this phase. This phase of expiration indicates a milder obstruction. However, if present during both inspiration and expiration, there may be more severe airway narrowing.

An absence of wheezing can be puzzling. It can indicate improvement of bronchoconstriction, but it can also result from severe and widespread airflow obstruction. For example, the tubes' airflow rates may be too low to generate wheezing, or mucus may be obstructing large regions of the airways. If this occurs, the person's lungs may tighten so much that there is no air movement to produce wheezing. This is called "silent chest" and is a dangerous sign and can lead to a severe condition called status asthmaticus, in which asthma attacks follow one after another without pause.

Asthma does not just happen and affect the person once or twice. In normal breathing, the distribution of ventilation and blood flow is evenly balanced, and the oxygen–carbon dioxide exchange is complete. However, if airflow obstruction continues, it contributes to physiological and clinical changes. The airway obstruction may be spread out and result in ventilation-perfusion inequality and hypoxia when body cells do not receive oxygen.

Another condition may also result when the person may inhale at high speeds. This breathing does tend to keep airways open, but it puts intense demands on the muscular work of breathing just to provide adequate ventilation. Most asthmatics complain of more extreme difficulty during inspiration than expiration because it is a lot of work to breathe through stiff, noncompliant lungs.

There are several explanations for the cause of bronchoconstriction and the airway problems in asthma. None thoroughly explain them, and some may interrelate or overlap. For example, one hypothesis relates to an immunologic reaction in allergic asthma. It involves essential biochemical reactions between an antigen and an antibody, such as immunoglobulin E (IgE), that binds to sensitized mast cells lining the airway and basophils. Strong biochemicals contract the bronchial tubes' smooth muscles, make the vessels more permeable, increase mucus secretion, and thereby attract inflammatory cells.

Asthma does not just happen and affect the person once or twice. In normal breathing, the distribution of ventilation and blood flow is evenly balanced and makes the oxygen–carbon dioxide exchange complete. However, if airflow obstruction continues, it contributes to physiological and clinical changes. The airway obstruction may be spread out and not uniform and result in ventilation-perfusion inequality and hypoxia (body cells do not receive oxygen).

Most asthmatics complain of greater difficulty during inspiration than expiration because it is a lot of work to breathe through these stiff and noncompliant lungs.

Nonallergic asthma involves another explanation. Stimuli such as exercise, infection, or air pollution provoke this type of asthma. Chemical or mechanical stressors stimulate the parasympathetic nervous system, specifically the vagus nerve (the longest cranial nerve that oversees crucial motor and sensory impulses). This stimulation causes the airway mucosa to overreact, leading to bronchoconstriction and wheezing.

SHORTNESS OF BREATH

Another symptom of asthma is shortness of breath, which combines with other symptoms. Wahls (2012) defined shortness of breath as a "subjective experience of breathing discomfort." He also outlines the following questions that a provider might ask regarding shortness of breath:

- When did you first feel short of breath?
- How long has it been going on?
- How do you describe it?
- Does it feel this way all the time, or does it come and go?
- What other symptoms have you noticed?

The medical term for shortness of breath is dyspnea. The word "dyspnea" comes from two Greek words, *dys*, meaning "with difficulty," and *pnoe*, meaning "breathing." When pronouncing the name, the "p" is silent.

The narrowing of the airways usually causes shortness of breath in asthma. One or both of the following reasons result in shortness of breath: muscles surrounding the airways tighten, called bronchospasm, and inflammation makes the airways swell and fill with mucus. The subjective evaluation of dyspnea includes a description of the person's hungry for air, rapid breathing, running out of air, or not breathing fast or deep enough. Like being hungry or thirsty, shortness of breath is impossible to ignore. The health-care provider cannot observe or measure it but must rely on the patient to describe the feeling.

If one exercises hard or has a cold and stuffy nose, some breathlessness is normal. It can also come on suddenly but disappear. In children, infections and upper airway blockage are the most common causes of breathlessness in asthma. The highest occurrence of breathlessness is in people who are 55 to 69 years old. However, shortness of breath that lasts for more than one month is called chronic dyspnea.

There can be many causes of dyspnea, including asthma, heart failure, chronic obstructive pulmonary disease, interstitial lung disease, pneumonia, or psychogenic disorders.

COUGHING

Coughing can be one of the symptoms of asthma. The main reason for coughing is to remove foreign particles and bacteria that gather in the respiratory system and prevent infection. Coughing is one of the body's natural defense mechanisms.

Coughs have two types: productive and nonproductive. A productive cough is one in which the person expels a noticeable amount of phlegm and mucus, enabling the lungs to rid itself of harmful substances. A nonproductive cough is a dry cough that responds to some irritant that causes the bronchial tubes to constrict. The airways swell and tighten, prompting the kind of cough that characterizes asthma. Often, wheezing will accompany this cough.

There is a type of asthma in which the primary symptom is a dry, nonproductive cough. Individuals with cough-variant asthma often do not have other classic symptoms such as wheezing or shortness of breath. This cough may last longer than six to eight weeks and can occur during the day or night. With this type of asthma, the person may notice coughing increasing with exercise or encountering such triggers as dust, perfume, or cold air.

Anatomy of a Cough

Why do people cough, and what causes a cough? The cough reflex starts when the cerebral cortex (the outer covering of the brain) transmits nerve signals through the vagus nerve. The vagus nerve is the longest of the 12 cranial nerves and controls the parasympathetic nervous system, which oversees the lungs and other organs. Along with the phrenic nerve originating in the neck (C3–C5), the vagus nerve passes between the lung and heart to reach the diaphragm. The diaphragm is very important in controlling breathing. It is a thin skeletal muscle located at the base of the chest and contracts when you inhale. This contraction creates a vacuum, and the air explodes into the lungs. When one exhales, the diaphragm relaxes, pushing out the air.

Lining the respiratory tract's epithelium are cough receptors that are sensitive to both chemical and mechanical stimuli. The bronchi and trachea are very sensitive, and the slightest amount of foreign matter can irritate and initiate the cough reflex. For example, stimulation of the cough receptors by dust particles produce a cough that removes the particles before they reach the lungs.

Coughing affects the diaphragm. Something stimulates the cough receptors that lead to exciting the phrenic nerve and other nerves around the lungs, creating negative pressure around the lung. Air rushes in to equalize the pressure. The recurrent laryngeal nerve tells the glottis to close. The glottis is part of the larynx in the upper respiratory system that holds the vocal cords and the opening between them. The vocal cords shut the larynx. Muscles in the abdomen contract respond to the relaxing diaphragm, and other muscles increase the lungs' air pressure. Now the vocal cords relax; the glottis opens, and air over 100 mph is released. The bronchi and portions of the tracheal collapse, forming slits through which the air is forced out and other irritants in the respiratory system.

Cough-variant asthma, in which the classic symptoms of asthma are absent, is quite a mystery. It could be that the coughing starts after people are exposed to allergens or breathing cold air. Coughing may follow an upper respiratory infection. For example, it is common to have asthma, along with sinusitis. Some medications, such as beta-blockers, may evoke a cough. Beta-blockers are drugs that treat heart disease, high blood pressure, and other conditions. These drugs are also found in eye drops to address common problems. These drops are associated with asthma cough. One who is sensitive to aspirin may also develop coughing with asthma.

Although most people connect coughing with the common cold or with bronchitis, it could be asthma. If the cough persists or lasts for longer than eight weeks, it could be a sign of cough-variant asthma.

CHEST TIGHTNESS

Classic or typical asthma includes the symptoms of coughing, shortness of breath, and wheezing. Another symptom experienced by some people is chest tightness or chest pain as a result of these symptoms. After an asthma attack, the airways may still be reeling from constriction and inflammation. Individuals need to be aware that this may happen and is relatively common after an attack. The person with chest discomfort should note whether their chest is sore or feeling a sharp pain.

Causes of Chest Pain

Because of the stress put on the musculoskeletal system during the coughing and wheezing associated with asthma, some individuals might experience chest tightness or chest pain. Taking a deep breath may cause pain. Also, after an asthma attack with classic symptoms, two medical conditions can cause chest pain, namely, pneumomediastinum and pneumothorax.

The mediastinum is the space between the lungs and other organs in the chest cavity, such as the heart. If the pressure increases in this area, a condition called pneumomediastinum will cause pain. The pain will usually radiate to the neck or back, and coughing, difficulty swallowing, shortness of breath, and spitting up mucus may also occur. The condition is relatively rare and will usually resolve itself. However, if people experience chest discomfort, they should seek medical attention because of the potential for heart disease.

A second condition is called pneumothorax, which occurs when a lung collapses and air leaks into the space between the lungs and chest wall. Symptoms include agitation, breathing fast, rapid heart rate, respiratory distress, and wheezing. A large pneumothorax can be fatal; hence, medical attention is essential if these symptoms occur.

NOCTURNAL ASTHMA

Nocturnal asthma is a burdensome symptom. Not only is it bothersome, but impaired sleep can also cause a host of other symptoms, such as daytime drowsiness and inefficiency. Although nocturnal asthma can affect people of all ages, the symptoms often start in childhood and are more common in children than adults. The AAFA sponsored a 2005 Harris poll that found 48% of child asthma sufferers experience disturbed sleep.

Why do some people experience nighttime coughing, wheezing, and breathlessness at night? Studies indicate that the relationship between nocturnal cough and impaired sleep is not clear. One proposal is that there is a circadian rhythm factor responsible for these nighttime disturbances. A circadian rhythm is roughly a 24-hour cycle in human beings' physiology, plants, and animals. This rhythm appears to be endogenous, although external stimuli, such as sunlight and temperature, can change the rhythm. Circulating hormones such as epinephrine, cortisol, melatonin, and neural mechanisms, such as cholinergic tone, may drive the circadian rhythm. Also, airway inflammation may increase at night, possibly because of a reduction in endogenous anti-inflammatory agents.

Studies to uncover the exact relationship of circadian rhythms have been inconclusive; however, many researchers believe that the asthmatic symptoms that occur at night are partly due to circadian rhythms. They use the term "nocturnal asthma" to describe the worsening of the signs at night.

Although not all people with asthma experience nocturnal asthma, those who do should take it very seriously. This condition is associated with more severe disease and increased risk of death. Those who have nocturnal symptoms should work out a plan with their health-care provider.

The Science of Nocturnal Asthma

Researchers describe that several mechanisms may make asthma worse at night. One of the main reasons is that whether a person sleeps or not, airway resistance increases throughout the night; the increased strength is much higher if the person sleeps. Another indication is that airway function is best just before the onset of sleep and decreases as sleep progresses. Thus, if a person with asthma gets a lot of sleep, the lungs' impairment will be increased. People with healthy lungs do not appear to have this problem; however, researchers believe that people with asthma frequently experience disturbed sleep.

FAINTING

The severity of the symptoms of asthma varies greatly. Fainting is one of the symptoms that are most severe and is one of the more extreme issues. Ignoring this symptom can be fatal.

The normal workings of the respiratory system is critical to good health and well-being. Asthma creates an abnormal condition by inflaming the airways within the lungs and chest, making it very difficult to get the right amount of air. Usually, bouts of these inflammations had previously signaled a chronic condition, but a severe flare-up can also occur, causing a situation in which breathing is limited.

When the brain does not get enough oxygen, fainting will occur. Unconsciousness occurs at first, and if the person does not get oxygen levels to the brain, he or she will experience brain damage or death. Fainting is the first stage of the condition, but it is an ominous sign.

BLUE LIPS OR CYANOSIS

One of the most severe symptoms of asthma is blue lips or fingernails. The condition is called cyanosis and indicated the lack of oxygen in the blood. When oxygen is present in the blood, it appears red; it looks bluish when oxygen is not present. With a severe acute attack of asthma, the cyanosis is sudden or abrupt, and the patient begins to turn blue because of the lack of oxygen. This occurrence is different from patients with specific chronic lung disease or COPD who develop cyanosis slowly over many years.

Again, this occurs relatively quickly. The areas around the lips and face are most susceptible to a lack of oxygen because the skin and membranes are thin in these areas. During a severe asthma attack, the signs of discoloration could be the blue tint on the lips and face; generally, the blue color goes away when the body restores oxygen, but on occasion it could be a prolonged issue. Regardless, the blue pallor needs to be considered a medical emergency and addressed as soon as possible to avoid serious complications.

FATIGUE

Fatigue is associated with asthma in many ways. Although it is not one of the more common asthma symptoms, it only makes sense to realize that when the body is working harder to breathe, one becomes tired. The body must compensate and bring more oxygenated blood from the lungs to the rest of the body, leaving one with a tired feeling. And even after a flare-up, the body may need time to recover to the normal healthy state.

Nocturnal asthma, with its consistent waking up during the night, can be characteristic of asthma. Getting inadequate rest and sleep during the night affects normal functioning during the day. The person is tired or exhausted. The stress put on the chest and lung area during coughing can lead to muscle fatigue and muscle pain. Constant wheezing can contribute to that feeling of being weak and tired. For some people, the feeling of being tired or exhausted can last several days after an attack.

COGNITIVE IMPAIRMENT

Although asthma primarily affects the lungs, it can also affect the brain and nervous system because of the effect on breathing and oxygen consumption. The increase of intermittent cerebral hypoxia in severe asthma is a factor. Some researchers have found the impact of asthma on cognition. For example, asthma may affect children in academic achievement, especially in the field of processing speed, attention, language, learning, and memory. Irani et al. (2017) performed a meta-analysis and review of studies done in the area of asthma and cognition and found several deficits compared to the performance of controls. In the study, 2,017 individuals were compared to 2,131 health controls. The cognitive deficits were global, with the most substantial effects on academic achievement and executive function. The severity of asthma was vital; the most significant deficiencies existed in those with severe asthma. The burden was highest with younger patients, males, people of low socioeconomic backgrounds, and racial/

ethnic minorities. The study concluded that asthma does affect more than the lungs. It creates a cognitive burden, especially among vulnerable groups.

DISORIENTATION

Another problem with asthma is that it may cause sudden confusion or delirium. The signs may vary. Some people become quiet and withdrawn; others may become agitated and upset. The person may seem groggy or dizzy or mumble things that don't make sense. This symptom is serious and calls for immediate medical attention.

EXTREME SYMPTOMS

Above, we have reviewed wheezing, coughing, chest tightness, and other symptoms. There are varying degrees of severity of these conditions. However, when any symptom becomes constant, the need for immediate attention is urgent. For example, if the individual is too breathless to eat, sleep, or do any daily activity, this is serious. If the person continues to breathe rapidly, this is serious. If the person feels his or her heartbeat is faster and continues for even a short time, he or she should seek medical attention. And if there is continued drowsiness, confusion, exhaustion, or dizziness, attention is needed. In summary, any symptom that becomes extreme and prolonged signals a need for urgent care.

CONCLUSION

Asthma is a common long-term inflammatory disease of the airways of the lungs. It has been recognized throughout history as a mysterious condition. The signs and symptoms of asthma are many. Some people may experience many or several symptoms; others may have only a few of the symptoms. This chapter discussed wheezing; shortness of breath; coughing; chest tightness and pain; nocturnal asthma; the effects of weather; and dangerous symptoms such as fainting, cyanosis, fatigue, cognitive deficits, and any signs that are sudden and extreme. Chapter 5 will consider how to diagnose the symptoms and also how to treat and manage them.

5

Diagnosis, Treatment, and Management

The symptoms of asthma are many. They can be very mild, requiring little or no medical treatment. They can be severe and life-threatening. How can one tell the difference, and how do health-care professionals diagnose, treat, and manage the symptoms of asthma? This chapter explores how asthma is classified and how strategies to diagnose children and adults may differ. We also discuss such diagnostic techniques as spirometry, skin tests, and the role of immunotherapy. We also explore various medications, delivery methods, and other strategies when individuals are not responsive to medicine.

ASTHMA CLASSIFICATION

Health-care professionals classify asthma according to the prevalence of symptoms, as presented in chapter 4. These types include mild intermittent asthma, mild persistent asthma, moderate persistent asthma, and severe persistent asthma. One must remember that these classifications are fluid, and people can move in and out of the various stages, depending on many factors. Although some doctors do not even use these classifications, they are effective strategies for helping doctors communicate with their patients to understand the nature of their conditions.

To classify asthma, doctors give a breathing test to determine lung function. First, a spirometer is a breathing machine that measures how narrowed the airways are. The second way of determining is peak flow that measures how fast you breathe air out, and if your lungs are working correctly. The doctor may then prescribe some type of medication to prevent symptoms and flares.

Although some children appear to outgrow asthma, the disease never goes away. The person just does not have an attack or flare-up. If one has a cold or flu, it can start up again at any time during childhood, including older years.

Intermittent Asthma

Intermittent asthma is occasional asthma, in which symptoms occur no more than two days a week. Occupational asthma, such as baker's asthma, is an example because the person may have the condition only when in the presence of a stimulus. If there are nighttime flare-ups, they probably never occur any more than two times a month. Although these attacks do not happen as frequently as other types, they still need attention and treatment. This type of asthma may include the classic symptoms of chest tightness, coughing, wheezing, and difficulty breathing. However, it often has little impact on one's daily life.

Mild Persistent Asthma

This type is the least severe of the four types of persistent asthma classifications. Individuals with persistent asthma may experience symptoms more than twice per week but not as frequently as once per day. The most common signs are coughing at night or during exercise or laughing, some difficulty breathing, chest tightness, or wheezing, especially when exhaling. Nighttime asthma appears to be a significant indication in determining the types. With intermittent asthma, symptoms may be no more than two times a month and no more than once a week. People may have flare-ups that prevent them from doing everyday activities, such as walking distances, climbing stairs, or cleaning the house. Still, generally, these do not occur enough for concern. Lung function tests show 80% function or higher.

Moderate Persistent Asthma

With this type, one may expect daily symptoms. Flare-ups can last several days. The person may cough and wheeze and not be able to maintain daily activities. Sleep is also affected. The lung function is about 60% to 80%.

Severe Persistent Asthma

According to the American Academy of Pediatrics, this type is the least common but more severe. Symptoms that arise throughout the daytime awakening impact sleep and physical activity. Lung function is at 60% or less.

DIAGNOSIS IN CHILDREN AND ADULTS

When diagnosing asthma at any age, some diagnostic strategies, treatments, and management methods may be similar; others may be quite different. For example, the doctor will take a current history, past medical history, and family history and perform a physical examination for both children and adults. In this chapter, we first consider children and adolescents and then look at adults. At the end of this chapter, we explain techniques, such as spirometry, immunotherapy, medications, and other strategies.

Diagnosing Children

After taking the child's personal and family history, specialized testing may be needed to rule out other possible causes of the symptoms. Younger children and babies cannot tell the doctor how they feel or if they are in pain, so it is up to others to describe the symptoms. Many children with asthma may appear and sound perfectly normal. A fussy baby could mean many things; toddlers may still be active even though their breathing is labored. Thus, the caregivers must describe the child's behavior, breathing patterns such as night breathing, response to medications, and triggers that may cause difficulty.

Young children may have difficulty in performing standard tests for asthma. For example, the spirometer is a device that measures the flow and volume of air blown in and out. Children younger than six have a hard time following the instructions to do this test.

Because the lung function tests are difficult to conduct with children, the doctor may see how the child responds to medications to improve breathing. The doctor may also order blood tests, allergy testing, and X-rays to get more information. A referral to a pediatric specialist or pulmonologist may be essential.

Infants and toddlers can use most of the same medicines as older children and adults, but the dosage may be lower and different. The drugs are usually given in an inhaled form. The doctor may recommend treating infants with a nebulizer (a breathing machine) or a mask with an inhaler or spacer.

After the diagnosis, the caregivers should plan for routine follow-up appointments with the health-care provider to review symptom control and treatment. Children should see the doctor for at least one to six months to monitor the treatment plan.

Diagnosing Adults

Adult-onset asthma occurs after age 20. Over half of the adults who develop asthma suffer from allergies. Occupational asthma, home environment, or polluted surroundings can cause the symptoms.

Adult-onset asthma can be quite complicated to diagnose because they experience many asthma triggers or have personal conditions. Hormonal changes in women, such as pregnancy or taking estrogen following menopause for 10 years or longer, can evoke triggers. Certain viruses, such as cold or flu, or exposure to environmental irritants such as animal dander, tobacco smoke, dust, or perfume can bring about adult-onset asthma. People who have gastroesophageal reflux disease (GERD) are candidates.

Because of changes in muscles and stiffening of chest walls, adults tend to have a lower ability to inhale and exhale as measured in tests. The decreased lung capacity may cause the health-care professional to miss a diagnosis of asthma. Therefore, diagnosing may be tricky, requiring special care. Several tests will help the doctor assess the situation. First, the spirometer measures how much air the person inhales and exhales. Then a short-acting bronchodilator is used to open up the airways, and the lung function test is repeated. If the spirometry test does not clearly show asthma, the doctor may recommend a methacholine challenge test, which causes the airways to spasm and narrow if asthma is present.

The strategies to diagnose asthma differ between adults and children. Many of the tests are quite complicated, and directions to follow are confusing, even for determined adults. If the child's diagnosis is asthma, the airways are sensitive and tend to stay that way throughout life. The symptoms may change over the years, and as children age, they may handle irritants better. However, about half of the children with symptoms will get them again in their late 30s or early 40s. New triggers may set them off at any time.

DIAGNOSTIC STRATEGIES

Asthma is not always a comfortable condition to diagnose. This section discusses strategies that the health-care professional may use in determining asthma. Some of the strategies can be used both for children and adults. The techniques include spirometry, bronchoprovocation, skin tests, FeNO, peak flow, and X-rays.

Spirometry Testing

Adolescents and adults can use this technique effectively. It involves following directions and a desire to cooperate to do one's best on the test. Children may have difficulty following the directions for this test. The word "spirometry" comes from two Greek root words, *spiro,* meaning "breath," and *metr,* meaning "measure." Spirometry is the name of the technique. A spirometer is a machine used in the technique.

Spirometry testing involves measuring the flow and volume of air blown out after a person takes a deep breath and then exhales. A person breathes into a tubelike device connected to a machine. It begins with full inhalation of an intense breath of air, and then the person is instructed to empty the lungs rapidly. Expiration is continued until a plateau is reached, and the efforts are recorded and graphed. There are four volumes of a person's lung function: expiratory reserve volume, or the additional amount of air that can be expired by determined effort after normal exhaling; inspiratory reserve volume, or the maximal amount of extra air that can be brought into the lungs by determined effort after normal inspiration; residual volume, or the amount of air that remains in the lungs after fully exhaling; and tidal volume, or the normal volume of air displaced between normal inhalation and exhalation with no extra effort. The reading of these four, added together, gives the total lung capacity (TLC). The measurements indicate various lung capacities, such as the functional residual capacity (FRC). Reading the forced expiratory volume (FEV) tells how much air a person can exhale.

Another important spirometric strategy involves reading the forced vital capacity (FVC), which is the total amount of air exhaled during the FEV test. To measure FVC, the person inhales as much as possible and then exhales as rapidly and thoroughly as possible. Healthy lungs can empty more than 80% of the air in less than six seconds. Forced volume expelled in one second is called FEV_1. A ratio is set up as FEV_1/FVC and expressed as a percentage. For example, FEV_1 of 0.5L/FVC of 2.0L gives 25%. The significance of the FEV_1/FVC ratio is that people with airway obstructions can be identified and also the cause of a low FEV_1.

Asthma diagnosis includes the FEV_1/FVC ratio. If FVC and FEV_1 are within the 80% value, the results are considered normal. The average values for the FEV_1/FVC ratio is 70%, with 65% in persons older than 65. In asthma, airflow is obstructed, showing a more significant decrease in FEV_1 compared to FVC. The score appears lower if the airways are swollen or constricted because of asthma.

Bronchoprovocation: Methacholine Challenge Test

A type of test called bronchoprovocation helps to diagnose asthma. This test involves asking the patient to inhale the drug methacholine, which causes mild narrowing of the bronchial passages. The methacholine challenge provokes bronchial tubes to narrow; thus, the name "bronchoprovocation" mimics asthma. If the challenge test causes a significant (20% or more) decrease in breathing ability from baseline breathing, it is considered positive. The positive indication suggests that the airways are reacting, and a diagnosis of asthma is possible.

One can get the challenge test in the doctor's office or a specialized laboratory. There are specific instructions given before taking the test. One cannot have food or drinks with caffeine or smoke six hours before the tests. Also, the subject can use no breathing prescriptions two days before the test.

Diagnosing with Skin Tests

There may be times when the doctor thinks a specific allergen is causing the asthma attacks and may request a skin test. Skin tests are usually quick and affordable and may give insight into the origins and treatment strategies for this type of asthma.

FeNO Test

This test is especially useful with eosinophilic asthma (EA), a type of asthma marked by high white blood cells called eosinophils. Nitric oxide is produced in the lungs when this type of allergy inflames the airways. FeNO refers to fractional concentration of exhaled nitric oxide and determines how much lung inflammation is present and how well inhaled steroids are suppressing that inflammation. The physician performs the test using a portable device that measures nitric oxide levels in parts per billion (PPB) in the air slowly exhaled from the lungs. This test is different from spirometry in that one must breathe slowly and steadily and not hard and fast. Some researchers believe that about 5% of adults with asthma have EA.

Peak Flow

The peak flow meter is a simple, inexpensive portable device that can measure how well air moves in and out of the lungs. Called "peak expiratory flow" or PEF, this handheld device can help one tell if asthma symptoms are in control or worsening. When one has an asthma attack, smooth muscles surrounding the airways tighten, causing the airways to narrow. The peak flow meter can alert the person hours or even days before an oncoming attack. This device is not so much for initial determining asthma but management.

Chest X-Rays

A chest X-ray does not reveal asthma. However, it can tell if something else, such as pneumonia or other obstruction, is present in the airways.

INHALED, ORAL, AND INJECTABLE MEDICATIONS

The best asthma treatment begins with a proper and thorough diagnosis. Many factors, such as the age of the person, severity and frequency of attacks, and understanding and following instructions relating to medications, are part of the diagnosis. Three components are involved in successful treatments: controlling and avoiding asthma triggers, regularly monitoring asthma symptoms and lung function, and understanding how and when to use medications.

Fast-Acting Medications

During normal breathing, the airways' smooth muscle system is very complicated. Local environment changes during breathing affect the contractibility, stiffness, and physiological function of airway smooth muscles. Local mediators, such as protein complexes, activate signaling pathways; environmental stimuli, such as extracellular matrix proteins, regulate the process. Pathological problems such as those created in asthma may alter the biochemical and mechanical action of the airways. A group of drugs called beta-agonists (B-agonists) affects the immediate issues of airway obstruction.

Short-Acting Beta-Agonists

As the name indicates, these drugs work quickly to control symptoms such as coughing, wheezing, or trouble breathing. These rescue drugs, called bronchodilators, open up and help relax the muscles of the airways.

The following is a brief description of the biochemical action. There are receptors called B adrenergic receptors; when these are activated, smooth muscle in the lungs relax, allowing the airways to open. A G protein of adenyl cyclase pairs with these receptors. G proteins are known as guanine nucleotides (one of the four components of DNA—adenine, cytosine, guanine, and thymine). G proteins, a family of proteins, are molecular switches inside cells that transmit stimuli from outside to the inside of the cell. Adenyl cyclase is an enzyme that produces a second messenger cyclic adenosine monophosphate (cAMP). In the lung, cAMP decreases calcium concentrations within the cells and activates another hormone, protein kinase A. These changes inactivate myosin light-chain kinase and activate myosin light-chain phosphatase.

B-agonists open calcium-activated potassium channels and airway smooth muscle cells. Combining the decreased intracellular channels, increasing the potassium conductance, and reducing myosin light-chain kinase activity leads to smooth muscle relaxation and bronchodilation.

There is a long list of B-agonists. In biochemistry, an agonist is a substance that starts a physiological response when combined with a receptor. Short-acting B-agonists (SABA) are the most common quick-relief drugs for treating asthma attacks. As of December 2019, four short-acting inhalers are available in the United States.

Albuterol. Albuterol is the chemical name of the first drug. Generic names are AccuNeb, Proair HFA, Proventil HFA, Ventolin HFA, and a generic solution for nebulizers. This medicine, which is in a class called bronchodilators, is used to prevent and treat wheezing, shortness of breath, coughing, chest tightness, and breathing difficulty. As an inhalation aerosol, it is used in adults and children four years and older; for oral inhalation, albuterol powder (Proair Respiclick) is used in children 12 years of age and older. Albuterol solution for oral inhalation (liquid) is used in adults and children two years and older using a special jet nebulizer, a machine that creates a fine mist. An aerosol or powder is used to prevent breathing difficulty during exercise and is usually used 15 to 30 minutes before exercise. Remember, albuterol only controls asthma symptoms but does not cure them; other medications work on pathological conditions.

Metaproterenol. This second drug relaxes the airways, preventing the symptoms of asthma. This medication comes as tablets and syrup to take by mouth and as a solution to inhale. As an oral inhaler, it is used every four hours to relieve symptoms or three to four times a day to prevent symptoms.

Levalbuterol (Xopenex HFA). This drug is another choice of B-agonist to prevent or relieve the symptoms of asthma. It is similar to albuterol.

Pirbuterol (Maxair). This drug is another choice of bronchodilator to prevent and relieve symptoms of asthma.

Long-Acting B2 Agonists (LABAs) and Combinations

LABA, a type of bronchodilator, lasts for 12 hours or more. The following LABAs are Foradil® (formoterol), Serevent® (salmeterol), Brovana® (arformoterol), and Performist™ (formoterol). The most common use of these drugs is in combination with an anti-inflammatory. The classic combination of LABA and anti-inflammatory medicines includes Advair® (Flovent® and Serevent®) and Symbicort® (Pulmicort® and Foradil®).

These medications work together. The LABA relaxes the airways' muscles, and the inhaled steroids reduce and prevent swelling inside the airways. The patient inhales these medications every 12 hours. Foradil and Serevent come in dry powder devices, and Brovana and Performist come in a liquid for the nebulizer. The combination appears to improve symptoms of those with moderate to severe persistent asthma.

Ultra-Long-Acting B2 Agonists

Researchers are investigating drugs that can last up to 24 hours. Refer to chapter 10, "Current Research and Future Directions."

Corticosteroids

Sitting on top of the kidneys are small glands called the adrenal glands, which produce certain hormones. Corticosteroids are a class of drugs that mimic the effect of hormones and, when prescribed in doses that exceed the body's usual production, can suppress inflammation. These steroids should not be confused with anabolic steroids that are taken by bodybuilders. Corticosteroids include cortisone, prednisone, dexamethasone, prednisolone, betamethasone, and hydrocortisone.

Systemic Steroids

Systemic steroids are those that are taken by mouth or by injection. For long-term asthma control, the doctor may prescribe oral steroids, which exist as pills, capsules, or liquids. These are not quick-relief medications but may be given for 7 to 14 days after a flare-up. The steroid drugs may control sudden or severe asthma and, in rare cases, long-term and hard-to-control conditions. Sometimes, they are used as a "steroid burst" for severe cases. Steroids and other anti-inflammatories work by reducing inflammation, swelling, and mucus production. These steroids include prednisone, prednisolone, and methylprednisolone. These drugs may cause side effects with long-term use. See chapter 6 for a discussion of the biochemistry of steroids and complications of long-term use.

Inhaled Steroid Medications

These medications are the mainstay for controlling asthma, reducing symptoms and flare-ups, and avoiding hospitalization. These drugs are slow-acting and can take effect only after several hours. Patients should take them daily for the best results. Some people may respond in one to three weeks, but others may take up to three months of daily use. The following are the most common inhaled steroids: beclomethasone dipropionate(Qvar), budesonide (Pulmicort), budesonide/formoterol (Symbicort)—a combination drug that includes a steroid and a long-acting bronchodilator drug, fluticasone (Flovent), and fluticasone inhaled powder (Arnuity Ellipta).

Leukotriene Modifiers

Research is occurring on a group of drugs called leukotriene modifiers. Allergens and exercise can often cause acute asthma attacks. Inflammatory molecules called leukotrienes precipitate these attacks. Mast cells release these substances, which appear to be the primary cause of bronchoconstriction. Eosinophils, a type of white blood cell, cause more severe cases of asthma. Leukotrienes and other chemicals attract eosinophils to the bronchioles. Scientists surmise that leukotrienes are critical in triggering acute asthma attacks and in the tightening of airways and mucus production.

Leukotriene modifiers are drugs that aid in controlling asthma by blocking the actions of leukotrienes in the body. The following are the Food and Drug Administration (FDA)-approved modifiers: montelukast (Singulair), zafirlukast (Accolate), and zileuton (Zyflo). These modifiers are taken as pills and decrease the need for other asthma medications.

Anticholinergics

Anticholinergic drugs block the action of the neurotransmitter acetylcholine and inhibit nerve messages for involuntary muscle movements.

They relax the smooth muscle in the airways, keeping them from getting narrower. They may also protect from bronchospasms and reduce the amount of mucus in the airways. The long-acting inhaled anticholinergic bronchodilators are tiotropium bromide, aclidinium bromide, glycopyrronium bromide, and umeclidinium. One of the most effective is tiotropium bromide or Spiriva Respimat, a long-acting anticholinergic used as a maintenance medicine when tighter control is needed. It is not a rescue inhaler and is recommended for children age six or older.

Immunomodulators

An immunomodulator is a chemical agent that modifies the immune response or the function of the immune system. For example, the modifier may stimulate antibody formation or inhibit white blood cell activity. Because many asthmatic conditions are allergenic and relate to the immune system, researchers have expanded investigation into this area of biologics in the past few years. This class of drugs is for patients with very difficult-to-control asthma. It acts as an add-on medication rather than a short-acting medication for acute relief. The following are approved biologic therapies: mepolizumab (Nucala), omalizumab (Xolair), and reslizumab (Cinqair).

The immunomodulator Nucala targets Interleukin-5 (IL-5), which regulates the white blood cells' eosinophil levels. This genetically engineered product keeps IL-5 from binding to the eosinophils, lowering the risk of a severe asthma attack. The drug is used in conjunction with other asthma treatments and injected every four weeks. Some patients experience fewer severe attacks and reduce the number of different medications. However, a few side effects include headache, swelling of the face and tongue, dizziness, hives, and breathing problems.

Xolair works differently from other medications in that it blocks the activity of IgE, a protein that some people with asthma overproduce. For people who have not responded to inhaled steroids, Xolair helps reduce the number of asthma attacks in people with moderate to severe allergic asthma. Xolair is administered by injection every two to four weeks but may have specific side effects such as redness, pain, and swelling at the injection site. It also carries a black box warning for potential life-threatening anaphylaxis.

Cinqair is also used with regular asthma medications when one cannot control attacks. It works by reducing the number of eosinophils. The doctor administers this medication as an intravenous injection for an hour every four weeks; side effects can include muscle pain, anaphylaxis, and cancer.

METHODS OF DELIVERING ASTHMA DRUGS

This chapter has focused on the diagnosis, treatment, and management of asthma symptoms. Methods of delivery have been alluded to for many of the drugs. This section focuses on the methods and types and discusses each one in detail.

Metered-Dose Inhalers

This system of delivery consists of a pressurized canister containing medication that fits into a boot-shaped plastic mouthpiece. Pushing the canister into the boot releases the medication. This method enables the drug to go directly to the airways and dispense liquid or fine powder medications, which mix with the air breathed into the lungs. However, there are a few problems. Proper use is essential. The inhaler should be shaken and then fired into the mouth after the start of a slow, full inspiration. The person holds the air for about 10 seconds. Almost a quarter of patients have difficulty using a metered inhaler. Older adults and people with arthritis may find it hard to activate the inhaler and can be helped by a device that responds to squeezing, called a Haleraid device. When used for children, a spacer and face mask ensures that the highest medication reaches the lungs. Although the patient may use the inhaler correctly, only about 10% of the drug reaches the airways below the larynx; the remainder may be swallowed and slowly absorbed by the gastrointestinal tract.

Breath-Activated Aerosol Inhalers

These metered inhalers are available for most classes of drugs. The valve on the inhaler is activated as the patient breathes in. This device requires a lower inspiration flow and is useful for those who may have trouble coordinating inhalation. Chlorofluorocarbons (CFCs) in the inhalers are pressurized and metered dose in a canister that contains a propellant. The propellant converts the medicine into small particles. The CFC evaporates before it reaches the lungs.

CFC-Free Inhalers

In 1987 participants signed the Montreal Protocol, a global agreement to protect the stratospheric ozone layer by phasing out production and consumption of ozone-depleting substances. The propellants in the old inhalers used CFCs and appeared to affect the ozone layer. New inhalers free of CFCs have hydrofluoroalkanes (HFAs or hydrofluorocarbons). HFAs are greenhouse gases, but they do not damage the ozone layer, which protects the earth from the sun's damaging ultraviolet rays.

On January 1, 2010, an amendment to the Clean Air Act outlawed CFC propellants used in most inhalers. Manufacturers ceased to make and sell, and even other countries began phasing out. People living with asthma were forced to switch to the more environmentally friendly HFA-propellant inhalers.

Many users began to insist that the new replacement inhalers do not work and might even be harmful. However, a spokesman for the American College of Allergy, Asthma, and Immunology said that sensation differences might have confused them. The mist feels softer than the CFC inhaler, tastes differently, must be primed before use, and must be cleaned more often. The less forceful spray makes people think the inhalers are not working. Most physicians say that it takes time for patients to become used to the new technology type, but the medication and effectiveness are the same.

Spacer Devices

A spacer device is a plastic tube with a mouthpiece or mask at one end and a space to insert an inhaler at the other end. Some individuals require help to use the inhaler. A spacer device is available to help that person effectively breathe. This tube attaches to the inhaler and holds it until one can breathe the medication. Spacers are especially advantageous for younger children or those starting out using an inhaler. One of the benefits of using a spacer is that it gives more time to use the inhaler and make the use much more uncomplicated. It eliminates the need for coordination when pressing the inhaler and breathing at the same time. Spacers extend the amount of time needed to deliver the medication and allow the lungs to absorb the medicine more slowly and smoothly. Although some spacers are built in, not all inhalers have spacers, so one should check with the pharmacist.

Dry Powder Inhaler

With this inhaler, one does not have propellant to push out the medication but releases it by breathing in a deep, fast breath. Some of the devices hold up to 200 doses, and others may have one dose that the user fills with a capsule before each treatment.

Researchers from Mayo Clinic have compared the three—metered-dose inhaler, metered dose with spacer, and dry powder inhaler—and encourage patients to find the one most suited for their needs. Following is the comparison. The metered-dose and dry powder inhalers are small and easy to carry; the metered-dose inhaler with a spacer is less convenient. The metered-dose inhaler, with or without a spacer, does not require a deep, fast, inhaled breath. The dry powder inhaler requires deep, rapid inhalation. With metered inhalers, with or without space, breathing out a little is not a problem; with the dry powder inhaler, breathing out can blow away the medicine. Metered-dose inhalers require one to coordinate breathing and medication release; metered-dose inhalers with spacer and dry powder inhalers do not require breathing coordination. Metered-dose inhalers and dry powder inhalers can result in medication depositing on the back of the tongue or throat; metered-dose inhalers with spacers allow fewer medication deposits on the back of the throat. Metered inhalers with or without spacers do not always show when medication is running low; with dry powder inhalers, one always knows when the medicine is low. With a metered dose, with or without a spacer, humidity does not affect the medication; with the dry powder inhaler, humidity may cause the medicine to clump together.

Nebulizer

A nebulizer distributes asthma medication as a fine mist that is breathed in through a mouthpiece or mask worn over the nose and mouth. Small infants or older adults who cannot use other devices may need a mouthpiece or mask.

Tablets and Syrups

For treating more severe episodes, tablets and syrups may work well. These steroid pills and syrups reduce swelling and mucus production in the airways. Common steroid pills and liquids include Deltasone (aka prednisone), Medrol (aka methyl-prednisolone), and Orapred, Prelone, or Pediapred (akaprednisolone).

Injections and Infusions

These drugs have been developed as biologics and used in immunotherapy. They act more like vaccines. For information on the current research and future directions and other strategies when medications are not working, refer to chapter 10.

CONCLUSION

This chapter has focused on the diagnosis, treatment, and management of asthma. We have discussed asthma classification and the differences in the diagnoses of adults and children. The chapter has featured tests such as spirometry and skin tests. We have described fast-acting and long-term control medications, along with their delivery methods. Chapter 6 focuses on the long-term prognoses in both children and adults and considers potential complications from the use of corticosteroids and other medications.

6

Long-Term Prognosis and
Potential Complications

LONG-TERM ASTHMA PROGNOSIS IN CHILDREN

The pediatrician diagnosed five-year-old J. J. with asthma in August 2019 and placed him on medication. One week in late November, he developed pneumonia, and his mom stayed up until 3:00 a.m. on Monday, monitoring his breathing and making sure pneumonia did not flare up again. She dozed off to sleep in a chair beside him, but he was not breathing when she awakened two hours later. The frantic parents called 911, but the paramedics could not revive him. The coroner told his parents that J. J. died of an asthma attack in his sleep.

His grieving parents said that he had not had an asthma attack in a month or more, and they thought he was getting better. But an asthma specialist told them how difficult it is to treat young children because they cannot describe their symptoms. And he added that asthma is very unpredictable, and it is unusual and rare, but severe asthma can happen at any time.

This true story from Colorado Springs illustrates that asthma is a severe and fickle condition. Likewise, the prognosis for any one individual is difficult. Childhood asthma often starts before school age. With these children, the lifetime risk is about 35%, with most cases occurring early in life and requiring lifelong medication.

In looking at the prognosis for asthma, the consensus among health-care professionals is that there is no cure for asthma, but there are treatments. Children with asthma can expect a life of caution, even though the attacks are not frequent or severe.

According to the 2017 studies from the CDC, more than 11.4 million people have asthma, including more than 3 million children who have had one or more attacks. This condition is the leading chronic disease in children and is more common in children than adults. About 6.2 million children under 18 have asthma; this figure reflects one in 12 children. Asthma is the main reason for missed school days. The last figure reported in 2014 was about 13.8 million missed school days due to asthma. Chapter 8 discusses the role of health education in schools and the importance of efforts to raise awareness.

The Prognosis for Children Younger than Six

How does one know if a baby, toddler, or young child is having an asthma attack? Asthma may have some of the same common symptoms, such as cough, sore throat, runny nose, nasal congestion, headache, facial pressure, and sneezing, as are present in many other conditions. A young child cannot talk about how he or she feels, and it is up to the caregiver to watch and determine. Close observation may give some clues. If the baby is panting or breathing rapidly during everyday activities that usually do not get the baby winded, it may be asthma. The child may gasp during normal play activities. Also, the nostrils may flare, and the skin around and between the ribs may appear sucked in. Exaggerated abdominal movement may occur. The baby may wheeze or make a whistling sound; however, some kinds of noisy breathing may sound like wheezing. The lack of oxygen may cause the child to exhibit a pale or blue face, lips, or fingertips. And of course, there can be a persistent cough that seems to occur most often at night or is triggered by play or cold air. Doctors can detect asthma only with a stethoscope.

A virus triggers most asthma cases. These cases are upper respiratory tract infections (URTI). Of infants who wheeze with URTIs, by age six, 60% are without symptoms. Those who have recurrent asthma by age six may develop airway constriction later in childhood. Asthma symptoms that start in childhood can disappear as the child grows; however, it may appear again in later life. Some children with severe asthma never outgrow it. Unless connected with a viral infection, children who develop asthma before age three have a poor prognosis.

Diagnosing a child under the age of six is difficult because they cannot perform pulmonary tests, such as spirometry. Instead, the doctor may try different asthma medicines to see how the child responds.

Health-care professionals do not know the specific causes of asthma in children. If the family has a history of allergies or asthma, the child is at higher risk. One of the most common causes is a respiratory virus. Both adults and children can get infections, but children have more of them. Some preschool children often get these infections, with at least half of children with asthma showing signs before age five.

Asthma in infants and children manifests differently than in adults. Because the airways are tiny, even very small blockages caused by viral infections, tight airways, or mucus can make breathing difficult. Detection is difficult because the symptoms are similar to other illnesses or diseases. The following conditions are nearly identical to asthma: bronchiolitis, croup, acid reflux, pneumonia, upper respiratory viruses, aspiration, inhaled objects, epiglottis, cystic fibrosis, or congenital disabilities.

For the physician, diagnosis is difficult for infants and toddlers. In a baby, fussiness can mean anything. On the other hand, toddlers and pre-schoolers may be active and running around even though they have trouble breathing. Lung function tests are hard to do with young children, so the doctor may order blood tests, allergy testing, and X-rays to get information. Often they give medications to see how well the child responds. The doctor may refer the child to a pulmonologist, a specialist who diagnoses and treats lung conditions.

Infants and children can use most of the medications prescribed for adults. The dosage may be lower, and the method of delivery may be different. Inhaled medicines appear to work well and have fewer side effects than medications taken in other ways. Medication given by a nebulizer or using an inhaler with a spacer and mask may treat infants. The delivery method called a nebulizer is a small machine that uses forced air to make a fine mist that the baby can breathe through a mask. Treatments may take about 10 minutes. The child may also use a spacer with a small tube that holds the medicine and is released as the child breathes in. In some cases, the child may prefer the inhaler with a spacer and mask.

Many medications are available to treat asthma; these may vary and smaller amounts prescribed for infants and children. Bronchodilators include ProAir®, PROVENTIL®, VENTOLIN®, and XOPENEX HFA®; these quick-relief medicines open up airways right away to make breathing easier. Long-term control medicines include inhaled corticosteroids (FLOVENT®, Pulmicort, Asmanex®, QVAR®) or leukotriene modifiers (SINGULAIR®); these medications calm inflammation in the airways and keep asthma symptoms low. Infants and toddlers may be given a mix of medicines, depending on how severe and how often they have symptoms.

There is a myth that children can outgrow asthma; the truth is, it remains for the rest of their lives only if they have sensitive airways. Asthma symptoms can change over the years, and as people age, they may learn to manage symptoms and avoid triggers. Yet, about half of the children develop symptoms again in their late 3s or early 40s. New triggers may set off the symptoms at any time.

The Prognosis for Adult Asthma

Although most asthma cases appear during childhood, it can arise at any age; when it first appears in adulthood, it is called adult-onset asthma. According to the American Lung Association (ALA), 1 in 12 adults has asthma and problems breathing.

The reasons that adults develop asthma are not clear. Many triggers are present, such as respiratory infections, allergies, smoke, mold, and many others. Why some people respond to the triggers and others do not is unclear.

Asthma can appear at any stage of life. It can develop at age 50, 60, or even later. According to the AAFA, about 50% of children with the condition appear to outgrow it when they reach their teen years only to have it reappear in one form or another throughout adulthood.

Because of their life experiences, adults are exposed to many things in their daily lives. If they exercise, they may have exercise-induced bronchoconstriction. They can develop allergies through life that could result in allergic asthma. Asthma and COPD can overlap. They may develop a nonallergic or even an occupational allergy.

Asthma in adults also can be challenging to diagnose. Early warning signs can be a frequent cough, especially at night; shortness of breath or panting; and frequently feeling tired. A chest X-ray does not show if a person has asthma but can show pneumonia or other obstruction. Often it is diagnosed in adults with their history and a physical exam. Several tests, such as spirometry, methacholine challenge, peak flow, or the exhaled nitric oxide test, determine the condition.

Stress appears to play a significant role in adult asthma. In adults, stress is a common trigger for asthma. When one has anxiety and asthma, they may feel shortness of breath, anxious, or even frightened. Chapter 7, "Effects on Family and Friends," investigates the role that stress plays in asthma.

Childhood and adult-onset asthma may share some things in common but also have some differences. The triggers may be similar, although different people have different triggers. Children are more likely to have intermittent symptoms with allergens setting off an attack because their bodies are still developing. In adults, symptoms are usually persistent and often require daily treatment. According to the AAFA, about 30% of adult cases are related to allergies. Women are more likely to develop the condition after age 20; obesity increases the chances of developing it. Deaths from an asthma attack are rare and then occur mainly in adults over the age of 65.

Likewise, treatment and prevention of both children and adults share many common strategies. Quick-relief and long-term control medications are similar for both. Individuals may take long-term medicines for many years; most children and adults take a combination of these medicines. Both children and adults need to have an action plan for their asthma. This plan should be written and kept in an accessible place for family and friends. Chapter 8, "Prevention," discusses these plans and gives specific instructions on how to create them.

OTHER CONDITIONS AND ASTHMA

Many diseases look similar to asthma, and persistent asthma can develop into other conditions. Several conditions, such as influenza and obesity, exacerbate asthma.

Asthma and Influenza

Influenza (flu) and the common cold are sometimes confused. Flu usually hits one suddenly, and the person begins to feel ill very quickly. The person experiences muscle aches, coughing, sore throat, and trouble breathing. One person described the feeling like being hit by a Mack truck. Flu commonly includes a fever of more than 100 degrees Fahrenheit and lasts three to five days. Extreme fatigue can last for weeks. Cold symptoms are usually milder and last for about a week. For people with asthma, both conditions deserve attention.

Flu can trigger asthma attacks and make the symptoms worse by narrowing the airways. When getting the flu, both children and adults with asthma are likely to develop pneumonia or other acute respiratory diseases. According to the CDC, 5 to 20% of Americans get the flu each year. Since the 1970s, between 3,000 and 49,000 people have died from the flu each year. People with asthma are at a higher risk of problems related to the flu.

The CDC recommends universal, annual vaccination to reduce influenza-related mortality and curb viral transmission. Especially at risk are young children, adults older than 65, and those with asthma. People with asthma should get the flu vaccine beginning in October, when flu season may begin. The season usually lasts through May, but some strains may be around in the summertime.

Asthma and Obesity

Many studies have shown a correlation between excess weight and asthma. Excess fat around the chest and abdominal region may constrict the lungs, leading to asthma development and worsening symptoms. According to the ALA, excess fat may lead to taking more medicine and even hospitalization. Also, fat tissue can produce inflammatory substances that impair lung function. Certain cardiometabolic risk factors, such as high cholesterol and diabetes, may contribute to asthma-related breathing difficulties. People who are obese are at the most substantial risk for susceptibility to allergens, chemicals, cigarette smoke, and air pollution.

The CDC has studied the relationship between asthma and obesity and found that nearly 39% of adults with asthma are obese, compared to 27% without asthma. Asthma rates appear to be rising faster among people who are overweight. Of all American adults, about 7% have asthma; among overweight adults, 8% have asthma. But among obese individuals, about 11% have the condition. Women with obesity had higher current asthma prevalence (14.6%) compared to those in the normal weight category (7.9%) and overweight category (9.1%).

The connection may start early. A December 2018 study in the journal *Pediatrics* found that in a study of more than 500,000 children, overweight children had an 8 to 17% increased risk of developing asthma. Obese youth in the study were at a 26 to 38% increased risk of asthma. Recent research also reveals that overweight children become overweight adults.

Losing weight can help reduce the risk of developing these conditions. Even the loss of 10 pounds can make a difference in asthma symptoms. Regular exercise appears to not only relieve asthma symptoms but also improve outcomes.

CONDITIONS THAT MIMIC ASTHMA

Several conditions can appear with similar symptoms as asthma. Only competent health professionals with a multitude of tests can determine the difference in some of these conditions. Also, some of them may exist, along with asthma.

Sinusitis

Sinusitis occurs when the small cavities around the nose called sinuses become inflamed. These open spaces fill with mucus, and drainage tracts become blocked. Symptoms include headache, pain in the sinuses, green or yellow mucus coming from the nose, loss of smell, toothache-like pain, and fever. Acute sinusitis can last days or weeks, and chronic sinusitis lasts for three weeks or more.

Health-care professionals refer to the link between sinusitis and asthma as double trouble. According to the American College of Allergy, Asthma, and Immunology, nearly half of individuals with moderate to severe asthma also experience sinusitis. Inflammation of an allergen or irritant may trigger both. Also, the constant drip caused by sinusitis may trigger coughing from the throat and aggravate asthma symptoms. If left untreated, symptoms can worsen and result in more severe cases of asthma.

Myocardial Ischemia

Asthma, caused by inflammation of the airways, has nothing to do with fluid in the lungs or heart disease. The term "cardiac asthma" describes a heart condition. In this condition, symptoms such as shortness of breath, with or without wheezing; cough; rapid, shallow breathing; increased blood pressure and heart rate; and a feeling of apprehension may occur. In the heart condition, one may notice shortness of breath first when the person is doing normal activities or lying flat in the bed. This disease is a heart function characterized by inadequate blood flow to the muscle tissue of the heart. The main symptom is pain, but the shortness of breath is another possible symptom.

Gastroesophageal Reflux Disease (GERD)

GERD is a condition in which the stomach contents and acid flow back into the esophagus, causing a feeling of heartburn. GERD can cause breathing difficulties such as bronchospasms and shortness of breath. When the stomach acid creeps into the esophagus, it can also enter the lungs, especially during sleep, and cause swelling of the airways. A study conducted by the American Lung Association Asthma Clinical Research Center found 38% of asthma patients have GERD.

Chronic Obstructive Pulmonary Disease (COPD)

COPD is a general term for several lung diseases, such as emphysema and chronic bronchitis. Over time, airflow is decreased, and tissues that line the airways are inflamed. Asthma, a separate respiratory illness, is sometimes mistaken for COPD because the two conditions have chronic coughing, wheezing, and shortness of breath.

Asthma and COPD may seem similar, but several factors demonstrate the difference. As people who have had asthmas as children, many lung disorders such as COPD may develop, People with COPD are adults over the age of 40 who are current or former smokers. The causes are different. There can be many causes for asthma; smoking or working in a highly toxic environment are specific reasons for COPD development. Both of these conditions are long-term and incurable, but the outlooks are very different. Asthma is more easily controlled daily; COPD worsens over time.

Congestive Heart Failure

Congestive heart failure occurs when the heart's left side does not pump correctly and causes a buildup of fluid in the lungs called pulmonary edema. The fluid causes problems during exercise with shortness of breath and even wheezing. With congestive heart failure, the wheezing is severe. The symptoms are very similar to asthma.

Bronchiectasis

Caused by repeated infections, this disease is characterized by injury to the walls of the airways. Clinical symptoms of both asthma and bronchiectasis may include cough, sputum, and difficulty breathing. Patients with severe persistent asthma may develop bronchiectasis.

Upper Airflow Obstruction

Some obstruction in the airflow may mimic asthma. Several conditions, such as enlarged thyroid glands or tumors, may restrict airflow and cause breathing difficulties. The tongue is a common cause of blockage in individuals who are suffering cardiopulmonary arrest. Other causes include swelling of the pharynx or larynx, trauma, a foreign body, or infection. Symptoms of airway obstruction are a change in the sound of a child's voice or cry, a cough, or gasping for air.

Vocal Cord Dysfunction

Dysfunction of the vocal cords is the abnormal closing of the vocal cords when you breathe in and out. Both asthma and vocal cord dysfunctions have similar symptoms: coughing, wheezing, throat tightness, and hoarseness. In the dysfunction of the voice box, muscles close rapidly, causing difficulty in breathing. Triggers can be reflux, airborne particles, intense emotion, voice overuse, cough, exercise, and fumes. Vocal cord dysfunction is sometimes misdiagnosed as asthma. Another condition may occur when there is a loss of function of the vocal cords; this also may be diagnosed as asthma.

Bronchogenic Carcinoma

This type of lung cancer starts in the lining of the epitheliums of the bronchus or bronchiole. Symptoms, which do not usually appear until the cancer is advanced, include cough, often with blood, chest pain, wheezing, and weight loss.

Aspiration

Aspiration is accidentally breathing particles of food or other things into the lungs. Acute aspiration may appear as coughing, wheezing, fever, and chest discomfort. Recurrent wheezing and asthma symptoms can be related to the aspiration of gastric contents.

Pulmonary Aspergillosis

One of the most common types of fungus is mold from the *Aspergillus* family. This fungus, whose spores are in the air, usually does not cause illness. However, those with a weakened immune system, damaged lungs, or allergies may be susceptible to developing the condition. Called allergic bronchopulmonary aspergillosis, or ABPA, the condition is a severe reaction to exposure to the mold. It is not common but can be a rare cause of poorly controlled asthma, occurring in less than 1% of patients.

Respiratory Syncytial Virus (RSV)

This virus can cause wheezing and pneumonia in babies and children. The connection of the virus as a cause of asthma is debatable. The long list of conditions can mimic asthma, and many are present, along with asthma. The possibility of asthma that is not carefully treated or ignored causes a risk of chronic lung disease in later life. According to the CDC, the person with severe asthma is 17 times more likely to develop emphysema, 10 times more likely to develop chronic bronchitis symptoms, and 12.5 times more likely to develop COPD.

COMPLICATIONS FROM LONG-TERM USE OF CORTICOSTEROIDS

The corticosteroids include cortisone, hydrocortisone, and prednisone. They are instrumental in treating many conditions, including asthma. The corticosteroids mimic the effects of hormones produced in the adrenal glands, small glands that sit on top of the kidneys. If they present over the body's normal levels, they suppress inflammation and reduce asthma signs and symptoms. However, they can also suppress the immune system, which controls conditions when that system mistakenly attacks its tissues.

Corticosteroids carry a risk of side effects, which can cause serious health problems. Knowing about these side effects gives patients awareness of steps to control the possible impact.

Side Effects of Oral Corticosteroids

When one takes a medication by mouth, the medication tends to affect the entire body and not just one particular area. Side effects depend on the dose of medicine. Therefore, three months appears to be the optimal time for the use of most oral medications. There is a long list of possible side effects that people who are using oral steroids should know.

Eye Disorders (Glaucoma and Cataracts)

Glaucoma is a group of eye conditions that damage the optic nerve and is caused by abnormally high pressure in the eye. First reported in 1950, researchers found that long-term steroid use increased intraocular pressure (IOP). Chronic administration of steroids in any form can raise IOP, resulting in steroid-induced glaucoma.

Cataracts occur when the lens of the eye becomes cloudy, and vision becomes fuzzy. Researchers have found that steroids taken as pills or delivered intravenously can increase the risk of cataracts. Also, inhaled steroids have a similar risk. People taking steroids should visit their ophthalmologist at least once a year, making sure to inform the physician of steroid use.

Fluid Retention and Electrolytes

Steroids cause a person to retain salt and water, which causes swelling in the lower legs and feet. The person can develop high blood pressure and lose potassium. People who note these conditions should limit their salt intake and consult with a dietician to increase the amount of potassium in foods.

Endocrine Disruption

Taking steroids over a long period (over three months) may disrupt certain endocrine glands and the hormones they produce. Other side effects of steroids on the glandular systems include suppressed adrenal glands; delayed menstrual development; changes in the menstrual cycle; increase in fat replacement, causing fullness in the face, back of neck, and abdomen, along with weight gain; increased blood sugar and diabetes; and mood changes such as euphoria, depression, and delusions. The person may tire quickly and experience loss of appetite, nausea, and muscle weakness.

There may be an increase in body hair and acne. The skin may become very thin, with a tendency to bruise easily and poor wound healing.

Increased Infections

Long-term steroid use may increase the risk of diseases, especially with common bacterial, viral, and fungal organisms.

Ulcers and Gastrointestinal Disturbances

Long-term use of steroids may cause gastrointestinal disturbances and ulcers.

Low Bone Density

When taken orally, steroids may increase the risk of osteoporosis, especially in the spine. These medications decrease calcium absorbed from food, increase calcium loss from the kidneys, reduce bone formation, and increase blood loss. People must take protective measures by doing weight-bearing exercise, avoiding alcohol and tobacco, and taking calcium and vitamin D supplements.

Side Effects of Inhaled Steroids

Inhaled steroids are the most effective class of medications for asthma. Oral steroids affect all body systems, but inhaled steroids absorb through the airways into the bloodstream with few side effects. Only if more medicine is needed is the risk of side effects increased. However, there are some side effects of note.

Fungal Infections and Hoarseness

When using inhaled steroids, some medication may be deposited in the mouth or throat, causing oral candidiasis or thrush. This medical condition is the result of a yeast-like fungus *Candida albicans* grows in the mouth and throat. Creamy white lesions appear on the tongue, inner cheeks, the roof of the mouth, gums, and tonsils. The lesions are slightly raised and have a cottage cheese–like appearance. The throat may become red and burn, causing difficulty in eating or swallowing. Using a spacer with or without a face mask, which helps deliver medication directly to the lungs, can usually prevent thrush. The person should rinse the mouth and brush the teeth immediately after using the inhaled product.

For people over 65, there may be an increased risk for glaucoma or cataracts with high doses of inhaled steroids or over several years. However, research studies generally show that low and medium doses of inhaled steroids do not pose a significant risk to vision and eyes.

Side Effects of Topical and Injected Steroids

Application to the skin can lead to thin skin, lesions, and acne. Injected steroids can cause temporary problems at the site of injections, including intense pain. This pain is known as a post-injection flare. Doctors usually limit corticosteroid injections to three or four a year, depending on the patient's situation.

COMPLICATIONS FROM OTHER MEDICATIONS

Leukotriene Modifiers

This medication category becomes an alternative to low-dose inhaled steroids in those with persistent asthma. Generally, they are not as effective. The leukotriene modifier montelukast or Singulair* is taken by mouth daily and is available as a chewable pill or granule that combines with food. Some studies indicate that there may be an increase in mood behavior or aggressive actions, headache, vomiting, nausea, and insomnia. These modifiers can also interfere with other medications that one is taking, such as theophylline or the blood thinner warfarin.

Long-Acting Bronchodilators (LABAs)

Long-acting bronchodilators, also called long-acting beta-agonists, have at least 12 hours of effectiveness than reliever medications. LABAs should be used only in combination with an inhaled steroid and never alone. Although these medications work by relaxing the muscles around the lungs' airways, they are not to be used as a quick relief therapy for coughing, wheezing, chest tightness, or shortness of breath. Examples of short-acting medications are albuterol, levabuterol, and pirbuterol. One must never stop or reduce any medicine unless directed by the health-care provider.

One large asthma study showed that more patients who used a LABA died from asthma problems than patients who did not use the LABA. The findings related to deaths from salmeterol and formoterol. Although this relationship needs additional study, the point is to use the medication properly to avoid risks.

BIOLOGICS AND SIDE EFFECTS

A biologic drug, also called a biologic, is a product that is produced from living organisms or contains components of living things. These drugs are created through biotechnology and include a wide variety of products from humans, animals, or microorganisms. As of 2020, the FDA has approved five biologics: omalizumab, mepolizumab, reslizumab, benralizumab, and dupilumab. Several others are currently in development. Omalizumab targets a specific type of protein in the blood called immunoglobin E, or IgE.

Overall, safety studies on biologics have shown few side effects. Some of the side effects include irritation at the injection site, coldlike symptoms, headaches, sinus infection, or fatigue. Users of omalizumab risk anaphylaxis, and the doctor may prescribe an epinephrine autoinjector in case of a severe reaction.

CONCLUSION

The prognosis of asthma is generally quite good. The consensus among health-care professionals is that there is no cure for the condition, but there is treatment. Children with asthma can expect a life of caution, even though the attacks may not be frequent or severe.

There are excellent therapies available, and control of asthma is generally quite easily achieved. It may take more work for some than others, and it does take perseverance in using the prescribed treatments. But in general, asthma is not associated with long-term severe respiratory consequences.

Although most asthma cases appear during childhood, it can arise at any age. When it arises in adulthood, this is called adult-onset asthma. The reasons that adults develop asthma are not clear. Many triggers are present, such as respiratory infections, allergies, smoke, mold, and many others. Why some people may respond to the triggers and others do is not clear. Asthma can appear at any time during life. It can develop at age 50, 60, or even later. According to the AAFA, about 50% of children with the condition appear to outgrow it when they reach their teen years, only to have it appear again in one form or another throughout adulthood.

As we age, all of us lose some lung function; our lung function at 80 is not what it was when we were 30. In asthmatics, particularly asthmatics who smoke, the lung function loss may be more rapid. And there may be some long-term consequences of asthma in terms of loss of respiratory function. This is one reason we are so adamant about individuals treating their asthma effectively and not worrying so much about some of the theoretical side effects of drugs, but instead making sure their asthma is well controlled. With asthma, smoking is a no-no.

Complications can arise from the long-term use of corticosteroids, which makes careful monitoring critical. At times, the person must, with his or her doctor, decide the benefit of certain medications over the risk of complications. But in general, with care and an action plan, people with asthma have a favorable prognosis. Chapter 8 discusses strategies for prevention and care and developing an action plan.

7

Effects on Family and Friends

Asthma is not just an individual problem. The stress of living with a chronic disease of any kind manifests itself among many other relationships. This chapter deals with issues that many people overlook when thinking of what one should know about asthma. First, we consider the emotional and social effects on the person with asthma by exploring the meaning of stress and how it compounds asthma effects. We then explore the toll asthma takes on parents, family, friends, community, and school.

EMOTIONAL AND SOCIAL EFFECTS ON THE PERSON WITH ASTHMA

As we have read in previous chapters, asthma has a dramatic physical effect on the person, but we must also consider the emotional and social impact on the person's life. When one has difficulty breathing or an asthma attack, the experience is physically devastating. Certain emotional factors, such as fear, stress, depression, and mood disorders, may emerge.

Humans have great imaginations. Many of these thoughts lead to creativity and innovation. However, imagination may have a dark side. It can lead to a fear of things that might happen. The dictionary defines fear as "an unpleasant emotion caused by the belief that someone or something is dangerous, likely to cause pain or a threat." Many people who have physical conditions or disorders experience an array of fears.

The nature of asthma and its unpredictability can lead the person with asthma to develop fears in some situations. For example: What if I have an attack when giving an important speech or going for an important interview? What if I have an attack when I am with someone I dearly care for or want to impress? What if it happens at school, and I cannot breathe in front of my classmates? The person's imagination then takes over, and fear that the incident can occur at any moment is on one's mind. It is common for people to be afraid of dying if one of the attacks occurs. Overcoming such fears depends on how well the person can accept the fear and plan a strategy to deal with it.

In 2018, Health Asthma and Asthma.net surveyed what it was like to live in the United States. The study found that although 26.5 million Americans live with asthma, many misconceptions about the condition and dealing with it still abound. The survey asked questions to over 800 respondents and revealed four things that people with asthma fear most. All four have a profound impact on how they view their conditions and rate the quality of life. The fears included affording treatment, ending up in the emergency room (ER), aging with asthma, and death.

Affording Treatment

A common concern for people living with any chronic condition, including asthma, is managing the costs of doctor's visits, prescriptions, and treatments. The survey found that 36% of the respondents said asthma had a significant negative impact on their finances. A significant theme was the fear of being unable to fill medications due to cost. Coping with this fear means that people may not build a nest egg for things like education retirement. Many responded that they were thinking about the whole area of savings; the money may have to pay for their medicines.

Aging with Asthma

Two million adults over 65 die with asthma. Some patients developed asthma symptoms in their 70s or 80s. Some had childhood asthma that went into remission and then reappeared later in life. The average age of people in the Asthma in America 2018 survey was 54 years. Many of the respondents had asthma for over 25 years. One stated that she had asthma for so long that their family and friends did not take it seriously.

Many respondents said they look forward and plan for the future and have fear and trepidation about aging. They fear that taking medications for so long may endanger their health as they age. Kerri MacKay, a writer and contributor to Asthma.net, cautions patients, caregivers, and physicians alike to understand the differences that older adults with asthma may experience in how their disease may look or respond to treatment. "The more we know about our asthma, regardless of age, the better equipped we are to share our experiences with our care teams and take the steps needed to feel better," according to MacKay.

Ending up in the Emergency Room

It is surprising to read that the fear that tops the list in the Asthma in America 2018 survey was the fear of landing in the ER. People with severe asthma (32% of the respondents) appeared to be most concerned. Their main concerns were ending up on a respirator and not waking up again. One feared the need to be intubated. Common also was the fear of the level of care in the ER. One person feared they would be brushed off.

Fear of Death

According to the CDC, 3,600 people died from asthma and its complications in 2015. People with asthma read these statistics and fear the worse. They fear getting colds or flu with asthma and dying. The latest data from this survey is available at *Asthma in America 2019* https://health-union.com/blog/asthma-and-copd-in-america-2019.

Stress

Stress is related to fear in that it develops over a more extended period. Defined as a physical, mental, or emotional factor that causes bodily or mental tension, stress can influence a medical condition such as asthma. Stress signs include depression or anxiety, anger, irritability, restlessness, feeling overwhelmed, unmotivated, or unfocused. Racing thoughts may be a continuous worry. A person suffering from stress may also experience memory problems and make bad decisions.

Asthma attacks are unpredictable. Because individuals cannot foresee these attacks, they are much more stressful than events people can plan for. The feeling that an event can happen at any time leaves a person in fear that he or she is always in danger. Stress then becomes a reality and works into a vicious cycle.

"Asthma is triggered by many things, and one of them is stress," writes Dr. Pramod Kelkar, a fellow with the American Academy of Asthma

Allergy and Immunology. He emphasizes how uncontrolled emotions work on the nerves and constricts the airways' smooth muscles, causing wheezing, coughing, and chest tightness. Asthma and stress work hand in hand in a vicious cycle.

These emotions include fear, anxiety, hypervigilance, loss of control, denial, anger, guilt, embarrassment, denial, anger, shame, and confusion. All these emotions can add to the stress—it is often difficult to unravel the connections.

Environmental stressors may affect morbidity through physical neuro-immunological mechanisms, which social networks, social support, and psychological factors affect. Wright et al. (1998) reviewed the role of these psychosocial factors in the beginnings of asthma. They propose links between behavior, neural, endocrine, and immune processes. According to the authors' review, this biopsychosocial model shows 1067 ways through which stress impacts asthma expression. Stress is associated with the sympathetic and adrenomedullary system's activation and the hypothalamic-pituitary-adrenocortical cortex (HPA) axis. This system responds to stress with an output of adrenaline (epinephrine) and noradrenaline (norepinephrine) hormones. This output leads to increased cytokines, causing inflammation that can affect the bronchial muscles.

Anxiety and Panic Attacks

For many people with asthma, fear and imagination lead to anxiety. Anxiety is defined as an extensive feeling or worry about an event or specific situation. Everyone feels anxiety sometimes during his or her life, and it is a normal reaction to stress. But one can become so overwhelmed that she stops taking part in regular activities; this is a red flag of more severe complications. These feelings can lead to a serious anxiety disorder called a panic attack, a sense of extreme terror when there is no real danger. Physical symptoms of panic attacks include shortness of breath, rapid heart rate, weakness, nausea, hot flashes, or dizziness.

Some individuals with asthma experience frequent panic attacks; this even appears in some lists of symptoms. Asthma attacks are quite frightening, and the person may become extremely scared during an attack, leading to the imagination that a future attack can cause one to panic. Women appear to be more frequently affected by attacks than men.

The psychological impact on the person's daily life can depend on many factors such as asthma severity, limitation of activities, social and family support, age when symptoms started, and how informed the person is about asthma. A study from Johns Hopkins revealed that asthma impairs patients' well-being and can significantly interfere with normal daily activities, such as work and school. This anxiety hits children incredibly hard; asthma is the second leading cause of limited activity in children. Missing school can hinder children's development and success in school.

Thomas et al. (2017) found that asthma is associated with subsequent panic and panic disorder in people at risk for psychiatric morbidity. The condition may worsen asthma. Panic may alter individuals' behavior, causing them to overuse asthma medications and lack of compliance with preventive and self-management. Hyperventilation is a common feature of panic and may result in bronchospasms from the airways' cooling and drying.

Depression, Mood Disorders, and Psychiatric Symptoms

When a chronic condition interferes with daily functioning for more than three months a year or causes prolonged hospitalizations, the person may experience more profound disorders. Asthma is a prototypical chronic condition that has been linked to mood disorders and anxiety. Characterized by variable and recurring symptoms, airflow obstruction, bronchial issues, and underlying inflammation, asthma has been the target of several studies investigating the interactions with mood disorders, depression, and suicidal ideation. One Canadian study found those with asthma at a doubled risk for one or more mental disorders. Depression and anxiety are associated with lower adherence rates to medicine and disregard for personal care.

There is a growing link between severe asthma and mental health. Although not completely understood, scientists have found that anxiety and depression result in increased symptoms, leaving them emotionally drained and unable to manage themselves.

People on certain medications may have more issues with mental health. Amelink et al. (2014) found that people with severe steroid-dependent asthma may have a 3.5 times higher rate of depression and two times higher rate of anxiety symptoms than nonsteroid-dependent people. This happening may be a two-edged sword. People need steroids for asthma control, but the use may lead to higher anxiety and depression levels. These people should have access to psychological-based interventions that address asthma control.

Limited studies have examined psychological-based interventions. However, there is growing support for these therapies to complement pharmacological treatments. A promising treatment is Cognitive Behavioral Therapy (CBT), in which the person explores how their behavior affects thoughts and feelings. Yorke et al. (2017) conducted a randomized clinical trial of CBT with 51 patients. The study assessed CBT's feasibility and acceptability for people with severe asthma and not to detect effectiveness. More studies in this area are coming.

How the child copes with asthma plays a role in how the person adapts to the disease. Coping skills divide into two categories: avoidance and approach coping. Avoidance coping distances the person from the stressor and does not solve the problem; the approach strategy strives to change the stressful event. Mitchell and Murdock (2002) examined the association of self-competence, asthma coping strategies, and asthma-related functioning in school-aged children with asthma. Thirty 8- to 10-year-old children and their mothers from inner-city neighborhood schools were interviewed. The analysis revealed that children significantly related to their understanding of self-competence. Higher levels of active and avoidance asthma coping strategies were significantly associated with higher participation levels in activities and recommended management behaviors.

Asthma and Cognition

Although asthma primarily affects the lungs, it can also affect brain function through direct and indirect mechanisms. Irani et al. (2017) conducted a meta-analysis of cognition in individuals with asthma compared to healthy controls. They extracted data on cognitive outcome measures and sociodemographic, illness-related, and study-related variables from studies reporting cognitive test performance in individuals with asthma compared to that in controls. They found that a cognitive burden associated with asthma exists, particularly among vulnerable groups with severe asthma. This burden was most significant among younger males, from low socioeconomic backgrounds, and racial/ethnic minorities. Effects were independent of whether the child was an adult, the type of study (whether norm referenced or control referenced), or reported use of oral or inhaled corticosteroids. This burden is probably due to the risk of intermittent cerebral hypoxia in severe asthma.

SOME TIPS FOR PEOPLE WITH ASTHMA

What to do about improving psychological health depends a lot on a person's age, circumstances, and life demands. There are some things that people of all ages can do—and should be encouraged to do. First, one should be proactive in taking care of oneself. Even young children can learn and be aware of what asthma does. Just knowing what can happen can help one be more in control. Facing your fears and feelings head-on can help you learn to cope. Help others understand asthma and how they can support you. In 2011, 1 in 122 people had asthma, so you are not alone. Having a support team is essential. Living a healthy lifestyle is important. Chapter 8 will focus on prevention and include more about developing this lifestyle.

EFFECTS ON FAMILY

When a person—regardless of age—has a chronic disease, such as asthma, the family's quality of life is significantly reduced. The chronic illness places a great deal of strain on the family's physical, emotional, and personal health—especially that of the parents. Although the impact is often for young children's parents, it may also extend into adolescent and even adult years. People realize that family relationship plays a central role across the life course. It is essential to consider all types of relationships— including parent-child, grandparent, marital, sibling relationships, and older adults' family care.

Parents

Diagnosis of chronic disease in children drastically changes the daily life of parents. They are the ones responsible for managing any unforeseen or sudden circumstances. Kieckhefer and Ratcliffe (2000) reported that parents of children with asthma experience spiritual and psychological stress, anxiety, worry, and doubt about their ability to manage extreme situations. All kinds of frightening scenarios go through their minds.

Mothers and fathers appear to adapt differently. According to Brazil and Krueger (2002), fathers tend to have less support from family, friends, and neighbors; they do not have help with strategies that maintain social support, self-esteem, and psychological stability. In most families, the mother tends to be the child's primary caregiver and endures the psychological pressures. Often mothers have difficulty helping the sick child adjust to the illness and the issues they must face in society. Kherirabadi et al. (2007) compared the prevalence of depression among mothers of children with asthma with mothers of healthy children. The researchers found a higher prevalence of depression among mothers of sick children. A study revealed 33% of mothers lost their jobs during the year of the study. Other studies showed that mothers of children spent fewer times with their spouses, had time management issues, difficulty communicating with others, high levels of anxiety and stress, and difficulty managing their child's illness. Also, the illness of a child can affect the marital relationship.

Siblings

The stress of living with a chronic disease reveals itself in many ways among the various family members. For example, people with asthma can become frustrated with their illness and all the work that comes with it. They may be more likely to get involved in fights or be less cooperative, or they may be stubborn, depressed, anxious, or withdrawn, which can, in turn, affect the family dynamics at home.

Siblings of kids with asthma may feel guilty, thinking that somehow they have caused the illness. They also may be jealous or angry because of the additional attention their sibling receives, or they may be afraid that they may get asthma themselves. Some may even feel embarrassed by the symptoms that their sibling displays.

Family members can also help each other's behaviors. They can encourage healthy behavior and assist in social control. However, the stress in relationships can lead to health-compromising behaviors and processes that impair immune function, affect the cardiovascular system, and increase the risk for depression. The quality of the family relationship can have considerable consequences on the well-being of all members.

Having asthma in the family puts the pressure mostly on the parents. They must achieve satisfactory control, not only for the child but also because asthma is disruptive to family life. Asthma in the family affects sibling relationships, the home environment, and the parents' lifestyle. Parents often experience proxy stigma on behalf of their children. They may have a concern about the children's career aspirations and future well-being. Therefore, they may begin to tightly control activities that may be beneficial to the child. The denial of activities may force the child to change his or her lifestyle to avoid or reduce allergic reactions. The child may not be encouraged to take play, study, or enjoy leisure time. He or she may spend lots of time in the health-care system; spending hours waiting for doctors or responses is often nerve-wracking.

Literature about the impact on families with a child with asthma reports findings similar to those of the impact of any chronic illness on the family. Murphy et al. (2017) reviewed 14 studies on observed family communication in families with the chronic disease compared with families with healthy children. The studies found that families of children with chronic disorders demonstrate lower levels of warm and structured communication and higher levels of hostile/intrusive and withdrawn communication.

Family Financial Burden

Asthma is the third most common cause of hospitalization and accounts for one-sixth of visits to the ER. In addition to the stress of these visits, the costs may also become a significant family burden. The economic cost of asthma (all ages) has been estimated to be $6.2 billion, including $1.6 billion for indirect costs due to children's missed school and $1.6 billion to $2 billion for direct medical costs for children aged 0 to 17. This burden adds to a decreased quality of life for children and their families, low self-concept, an increase in mortality, and high costs for society. Estimates are that health-care expenditures for asthma in developed countries are 1% to 2% of all health-care costs.

EFFECT OF ASTHMA IN SCHOOL

According to the CDC, approximately 9% of U.S. children have asthma; according to the district and area, rates may range from 25% to 50%. In a classroom of 30 children, about three are likely to have asthma. As the leading chronic illness among children and adolescents in the United States, it is one of the leading causes of school absenteeism. Low-income children, especially those living in inner cities, experience more emergency department visits, hospitalizations, and deaths due to asthma than the general population. Boys are more likely to have asthma than girls.

If asthma is poorly controlled and cared for, symptoms can negatively affect school performance and disrupt the entire classroom. Children with poorly managed asthma may have more emotional, social, or behavioral problems, which hinders school progress. A host of negative things may happen. Both daytime and nighttime asthma symptoms can result in sleep disruptions, insufficient attention in class, failure to study at home, and limited participation in critical social and physical activities. One study showed that children with asthma are absent from school two weeks across the academic year; this absence period may be longer for children with extremely severe asthma.

Carrying inhalers at school can be problematic. Some schools ban them for good reasons. They fear lawsuits if children overuse the inhalers by huffing on them many times during the school day. Children may let others handle the inhalers, risking adverse reactions in other children. Some schools have a policy that students can only use medical devices in a nurse's office.

According to the clinical guidelines of the National Heart, Lung, and Blood Institute (NHLBI, 2007), children should attend school if their symptoms lessen with the use of as-needed medication. Still, many parents are often unsure when to send their children to school. The fear of a child having an attack in school complicates the decision. Also, if the child has had issues at night, the parents may feel that he or she needs to rest in the morning. The children themselves may be anxious about going to school. Fear of participating in physical activity may cause them to request to sit out an activity. Over time, this may reflect on their self-esteem, social interactions, and physical functioning. Rates of overweight and obesity appear especially in urban children because of the lack of physical activity.

Mitchell (2015) participated in an NIH-funded longitudinal study to assess the relationship of asthma and academic performance in a sample of urban children with persistent asthma compared to a group of healthy urban peers. They used objective and electronic monitoring devices in real time to examine children's experience of asthma, sleep, and school performance. They found that more asthma symptoms were associated with lower academic performance, such as grades, quality of schoolwork, and ability to focus in the classroom. The study associated poorer-quality sleep of shorter duration and disruptive sleep with poorer asthma management and more unsatisfactory school performance. Also, they found that those with poorer asthma management plus allergic rhinitis (an upper airway disease with symptoms such as sneezing and runny nose, which affects about 80% of children with asthma) had an increased risk for low school functioning. Of course, adherence to medications and reasonable trigger control can decrease these occurrences. However, medication adherence appears to be challenging for most families. According to the study, in ethnic groups, children tend to take their daily controlled medications around 50% of the time. The rate is lower in minority families. The families' knowledge of the benefits of medicines and concerns about their safety and effectiveness are factors that challenge the consistent use of medications.

There are many problems for children with asthma in school. The schools may have or may not have nurses or even people trained to care for children with asthma. Schools may not have action plans. Caregivers may not provide information about the child or communicate with the school regarding effective ways to control the child's asthma. The children themselves may not know what to do with their asthma symptoms, or they may ignore the signs. Their peers do not know what asthma is or how to support them; this can make them reluctant to take their meds in front of their classmates.

The poor structural and environmental conditions of some schools may harbor allergens. There may be pests, molds, and other irritants such as perfumes and strong smells. Children may be exposed to secondhand smoke at home and wear clothing exposed to tobacco smoke. Besides, teachers themselves may be unfamiliar with asthma and its symptoms and may not know about the child's treatment plan.

EFFECT OF ASTHMA ON SOCIETY

Although asthma may affect individuals, families, and institutions, asthma also has a significant impact on society in general. According to a study by Nunes et al. (2017), both the prevalence and incidence of asthma have been increasing worldwide in recent decades. The umbrella term "modern lifestyle" includes genetic background and a large number of environmental risk factors. Worldwide economic globalization may have also contributed to the increase in the burden even in countries that previously had a low prevalence of the disease. Nunez analyzed asthma as a global disease; asthma's burden, mortality, characterization, and comorbidities; international direct and indirect costs; and the social impact of asthma.

Recent data from the general population showed that in children up to 5 years old, the incidence rate was 23/1,000 children per year; among youth ages 12 to 17, it was 4.4/1,000 per year. Adult females had 1.8 times greater asthma incidence than adult males.

Although it may be a little-known fact, nearly 3,500 people in the United States die from asthma each year. The prevalence is exceptionally high among children, and it is also multiplying. Almost one in nine children in the United States has asthma. In the United States of America (USA), per the National Health Interview Survey (NHIS)-2012, about 40 million people suffered from lifetime asthma (13% of the U.S. population), and 26 million people (8%) had current asthma. The lifetime asthma prevalence in different countries ranges from 1% to 18% of the general population.

The socioeconomic impact of the disease focuses on evaluating the development communities have on social and economic well-being: changes in community resources, housing, employment and income, market effects, public services, and community qualities determine these factors. Nunez studied the country gross domestic product (GDP), geographic and demographic status, type of health system, organization of health services, primary care, hospital network, private clinics, financial resources on public health, prevention and promotion in quality of life, links with schools, pharmaceutical industry, rehabilitation of asthma patients and their work, generic drug availability for treatment, and methodology of collecting data.

The assessment of all this data of asthma burden is a challenge. Even when using similar research protocols, reports on asthma prevalence and disease characterization have shown significant disparities.

Costs to the families are high, but the average cost to society is over $50 billion per year in health-care expenses, missed school days, missed workdays, and early death. Although the figures are high among children, most asthma sufferers are over 65. It contributes to physical deterioration and even death among the elderly. Even the best treatments control some patients' disorders, and others may be completely resistant to all current therapies.

PSYCHOLOGICAL AND EMOTIONAL EFFECTS OF ASTHMA: TEDDY ROOSEVELT

He was known as a tough man, leading the troops in the Spanish-American War up San Juan Hill. He was a rugged outdoorsman. He was the 26th president of the United States. He also had asthma. Some historians think that his severe asthma shaped his many accomplishments.

Theodore (Teddy) Roosevelt was born in October 1858 to a well-known, distinguished family. He was a sickly child and could not participate in a lot of activities like playing outside or even going to school. He had many disabilities. In addition to debilitating asthma, he suffered from headaches, toothaches, and abdominal pain. His parents were very supportive and took him to many doctors to find help. Doctors in the late 19th century did not know anything about asthma. They suggested vacations to the coast, drinking coffee, and whiskey and the favorite treatment of the day: smoking cigars. None of these helped his condition.

Although he was confined indoors, his parents kept him busy. He had private tutors and wrote down all his experiences and thoughts in a journal. His parents encouraged him to read. When he went outdoors, he loved to collect and study plants and animals.

He was extremely close to his father, Theodore Sr., who took him on nighttime carriage rides to distract his son from his illness. He also built him a home gym, which included weights and gymnastics. Theodore Sr. lectured him on the importance of developing his body, mind, and heart. Dad also made it possible for him to ride horseback, swim, wrestle, box, and learn judo. Teddy also contributed his success to the exercise of body and mind to overcome asthma. He went on to Harvard University and ultimately to be president of the United States, always remembering his family's advice and support.

CONCLUSION

The psychological and social effects on family and friends are often forgotten in the hustle and bustle of dealing with this disease. It is not a one-person problem and manifests itself among many other relationships. The person with asthma may endure severe psychological issues that are not related to the disease. These issues of stress and fear can even morph into severe mental illness. The same type of stress and fear can develop in family, friends, and caregivers. The social ramifications are worldwide. Chapter 8 explores how the condition may be prevented or detected at the first opportunity to prevent future issues.

8

Prevention

Worldwide populations have seen an increase of both prevalence and incidence of asthma in recent years. The increase is due to a wide number of environmental and lifestyle risk factors. Prevention and early detection are topics that are of essential interest to not only individuals but to society. This chapter on prevention or early detection examines such topics as practicing good personal care, vaccines, lifestyle changes, asthma action plans, and genetic screenings. It will also explore how schools and communities can assist in prevention and care.

PRACTICING GOOD PERSONAL CARE

For those with asthma, knowing the triggers and how to prevent them is essential. It is gratifying to know that there are simple steps that you can take to prevent infections that trigger asthma symptoms. The CDC has published a list of actions for good hygiene and personal care.

Hand-washing

Soap and water are the best ways to reduce germs that will cause infections, which people with asthma must avoid. Always wash hands before, during, and after preparing food; before eating food; after using the toilet;

after changing diapers or cleaning up a child who has used the toilet; before and after caring for someone who is sick; after blowing your nose, coughing, or sneezing; and after touching garbage. If there is a disease outbreak in the community, stay home as much as possible; if you go out in public, avoid crowds and people who are sick. Be sure to wash hands when you return home. If someone in your house is sick, stay away from them and especially avoid sharing personal items such as cups and towels.

Aiello et al. (2008) studied the effect of hand hygiene on communities. They found feces on the hands from people or animals, which is a source for not only *Salmonella, E. coli 0157, but also for* noroviruses that causes diarrhea and can spread serious respiratory infections. A single gram of human feces, which is about the weight of a paper clip, can contain one trillion germs. Handwashing is so important because people frequently touch their eyes, nose, and mouth with their hands. The face is an area that one touches often without realizing it. Germs on unwashed hands can get into the body through these venues. The researchers also found that handwashing could reduce respiratory illnesses like colds in the general population by 16% to 21%. People with asthma may at some time need antibiotics. Handwashing helps battle the rise in antibiotic resistance, reducing about 20% of respiratory infections.

Cleaning and Disinfecting

You and your family frequently touch many things: tables, doorknobs, light switches, countertops, handles, desks, phones, remotes, keyboards, toilets, faucets, and sinks. When cleaning, do not overlook these items. The EPA is aware that people who have asthma or other respiratory illnesses can react to exposure to disinfectants. They recommend that one should always follow the instructions on the label and use only the recommended amounts. Use products that reduce inhalation exposure such as wipes or dampened towels. And be sure to wash hands thoroughly after using these products.

Disinfectants should be used, but avoid disinfectants that can cause an asthma attack. In fact, it is a good idea to have someone who does not have asthma clean and disinfect. Be sure to apply the disinfectant to a cloth or paper towel, rather than spraying it into the air.

Avoid Sinus Infections

According to the AAFA, half the people with moderate asthma have sinusitis. Sinuses are hollow places in the skull. They are connected to nasal passages and help moisten, warm up, and filter air as you breathe it in. Infections are usually caused by a virus but after a while can also be invaded by bacteria. Having both of these conditions can be a double-edged sword and, without treatment, can last for months. Sinus infections can make asthma more difficult to control. One avoids sinus infections by avoiding those with colds and viruses; this makes handwashing and personal hygiene very important. There is good news. Sinus infections have lots of treatments available; the key is treating the condition aggressively.

Developing Good Sleep Habits

Breathing disorders during sleep have many consequences, the most prevalent being daytime sleepiness and drowsiness, fatigue, and cognitive impairment. Sleep and night control of asthma is extremely important. The CDC has established some tips for getting a good night's sleep. Try to develop specific bedtime rituals and adhere to them. Do not go to bed until you are tired and do not watch TV, read, or eat in bed. It is a good idea not to engage in strenuous exercise or activity before bed. Avoid caffeine in coffee, tea, or sodas. Try to go to bed and get up at the same time, even on the weekends.

Sleep position may be important. It is suggested that you lie on our side with a pillow between your legs and head elevated with pillows. When lying on the back, try to keep the back straight with the head elevated and knees bent—perhaps a pillow under the knees.

Eating a Healthy Diet

Current research has shown a correlation between asthma and diet. Certain foods, including fruits, vegetables, whole grains, and other high-fiber foods, are beneficial, while others such as dairy products and foods high in saturated fats can be harmful. Alwarith et al. (2020) analyzed nutrition studies relating to diet and asthma. They found evidence suggesting that diets emphasizing the consumption of plant-based foods might protect against the development of asthma and improve symptoms by affecting inflammation, oxidation, and microbial composition. Increased fruit and vegetable intake, reduced animal products consumption, and weight management may mediate cytokine release, free radical damage and immune responses.

Fruits and vegetables may be especially beneficial and has been linked to decreased risk for asthma in children and adults. These have been shown to improve lung function and make asthma symptoms such as wheezing more manageable. Likewise, dairy consumption can raise the risk for asthma and worsen symptoms, according to the study.

Getting Proper Vaccines

It is also essential to get proper vaccines. Talk with your health-care provider about getting a flu shot every year. In addition, you may need a pneumococcal vaccine to target the common cause of pneumonia, an illness that can be devastating to people with asthma.

Two types of flu vaccines—a shot and a nasal spray—are available. Both kinds work the same way with everyone by aiding in the development of antibodies. Flu shots do not have a live virus and cannot cause the flu. People with asthma should not get Flumist, as it does contain weakened viruses.

LIFESTYLE CHOICES

Some psychologists recommend that you can remember good lifestyle development with the word NESS: N—nutrition; E—exercise; S—social contact; S—support system.

Maintain a Healthy Body Weight

This is very difficult for many people, especially in the days of fast food and advertisements promoting the Western diet. According to the CDC, 38% of adults in the United States are obese. The normal range for the body mass index is 18.5–24.9, with overweight being 25–29.9. This is not only a problem for adults but also children; 21% of youth between the ages of 12 and 19 are dealing with obesity.

The figures are especially important for people with asthma. Those with a BMI of 30 or more have a much higher risk of having asthma and managing symptoms. Seven percent of adults in the normal range have asthma, but 11% with the higher BMI have asthma. It is not clearly understood why women are especially at risk. Nearly 15% of those who are obese suffer from the condition.

Why does carrying extra weight cause asthma? Researchers are not exactly clear. Carrying extra fat around the chest and abdomen constricts the lungs and makes breathing more difficult. However, fat tissue may make things more complicated. In a research study, Dixon and Poynter (2016) found that the majority of patients with severe or difficult-to-control asthma in the United States are obese. Because obesity is a disorder of metabolism and energy regulation, processes fundamental to the function of every cell and system within the body, including the lungs, are affected. They propose in the study that reduction of obesity could help with lung function.

People with a BMI over 30 also do not respond in the same way to medications as people with lower BMIs. According to the American Lung Association, obese people have less asthma control when treated with theophylline, a drug used for relaxing bronchial smooth muscle. Other research groups have reported that obesity reduces the effectiveness of medications such as inhaled corticosteroids.

Obesity may relate to many conditions. People with a BMI over 30 tend to have depression and obstructive sleep apnea. They also may find it challenging to exercise or do simple daily tasks that involve movement.

CBT is a psychological strategy that seeks to change people's attitudes and their behavior by focusing on the person's thoughts, images, beliefs, and attitudes and how these processes relate to the person's behavior. Bazhora (2020) studied the effects of CBT in 78 patients with uncontrolled bronchial asthma against the background of excess body weight and obesity. When responding to the questionnaires, the patients had significant positive dynamics relating to emotions, activity, overcoming depressive disorders, and overall quality of life. Also, the nature of the therapy assisted in reducing the frequency of use of short-acting β-2-agonists, nocturnal symptoms of asthma, and use of oral steroids.

Increase Exercise

The right kind of physical exercise is an important strategy for preventing or minimizing asthma. Following are some of the benefits of exercise: increased endurance and building up tolerance, decreased inflammation of airways by reducing inflammatory proteins, strengthening muscles, and improved cardiovascular fitness.

The best exercises are low-density, involving brief bursts of exhaustion. Such exercises do not tire the lungs and are therefore suggested for asthma. Swimming is the most suggested exercise for asthma because of constant pressure on the chest; moist, warm air; and reduced pollen. However, chlorinated pools may trigger some asthma symptoms. Walking is a low-intensity exercise but should be done in warm weather as dry, cool air can trigger symptoms; you can also walk on a treadmill or indoor track. Hiking is good, but watch the pollen count. Recreational biking is a low-impact activity; you can also use an indoor bike. If you like to run, choose short-distance activities such as sprints; long-distance running is not recommended. Some sports fit in this category: baseball, gymnastics, volleyball, golf, or football.

Managing Stress

Chapter 7 examined in detail the effects of stress on people with asthma. Stress can come from worry, fear of what could happen, or from lifestyle situations. Children and adults may approach the problem of stress differently; yet, the same principles can apply.

Relaxation exercises combine deep breathing, releasing muscle tension, and clearing negative thoughts. Exercises may vary, but the following is an example of managing stress with asthma. For two minutes, concentrate your thoughts on yourself and breathe slowly. Scan the body, noticing the areas that are tense. Rotate your head in a smooth, circular motion, but stop if any movements cause pain. Roll the shoulders back and forth. Focus on pleasant thoughts and not negative ones. Remember, strong emotions can trigger an asthma attack. Be responsible for helping yourself cope with stress and anxiety.

Seeking Support

Remember that you are not alone. Accept the fact that life is tough, and support is the single most important cushion against stress. However, you should remain active and independent as much as possible.

Support can come in many ways. It can be a network of people—family, friends, or colleagues—who formally and informally provide assistance with a variety of needs a person has. What is important is connecting with other people with asthma. Formal groups are sometimes called "support groups" or "self-help groups." Each person's support system will vary greatly and depend on the individual's developmental level, life circumstances, and needs. Social support is important for stress reduction by having others share our experiences, concerns, or fears can help one adjust to the chronic condition and realize they are not alone.

Avoiding Irritants

You will be developing an asthma action plan but first you must learn about the triggers and some do's and don'ts. Sometimes these triggers will come from unexpected sources.

Aromas and Fragrances

It is important to know that there are two families of fragrances: those that occur naturally and those that are created artificially. Many people have asthma attacks from artificial fragrances. Knowing these triggers and how to avoid is important for prevention. Fragrances that cause the most problems are those that have many additives.

Perfumes are probably the most common. Although they are generally made with essential oils of natural scent, they have other agents to strengthen the fragrance and help it bond to what it is sprayed on. Common bonding agents are petrochemicals, alcohols, coal, and coal tar. Fragrances that appear to have little effect are those that are simple in their processing. For example, rose water is made with rose essential oils and water. It is also delivered with a spray from a pump bottle, rather than a pressurized aerosol can.

Aerosol delivered sprays, such as body sprays and certain deodorants, are delivered with force of air, and the scents are often artificially created aromatic chemicals. Bathroom sprays and air fresheners contain many of these same additives and make the air less safe to breathe.

Avoiding these harmful fragrances does require some knowledge of products. The idea is to look for simplicity. Take the time to read labels of ingredients. You should be able to read the list in 10 seconds or less. Simple products exist in every category: perfume such as rose water, sprays, deodorant, air fresheners, shampoos, soaps, and toothpaste.

Some offices will have notices posted not to wear perfumes in the office. However, if you are in a place where the perfume is strong, it is always important to carry a rescue inhaler.

OTHER IMPORTANT THINGS TO KNOW

Being aware of various aspects of asthma and its treatment can help an individual prevent asthma attacks, minimize their severity, or prevent long-term complications.

Risk of Corticosteroids

Use of corticosteroids is one of the topics that will be considered in chapter 9, "Issues and Controversies." You may find it necessary to use these medications. However, you can be aware of the benefits and risks of this drug.

Medication Sharing

Medications are individual and designed only for the use of one person. Do not share asthma medication or equipment. Others must not share any equipment such as an inhaler, nebulizer, or tubing and mouthpiece. But is this always the rule? Recently, officials at a Texas middle school suspended two girls because one loaned her inhaler to another. According to the recommendations of the American Academy of Pediatrics, schools should immediately confiscate medications when students share and take away the privilege of self-administering medicine. But what about when it can save a life? One doctor from the American College of Asthma, Allergy, and Immunology said that good sense sometimes trumps a rule. If a person is dying, then the medication should be shared. But it is not a good idea because all inhalers are not created equal; sharing would be an extreme instance.

Understand Asthma and Humidity

Humidity is the percentage of water in the air, compared to the amount of water the air can hold at a given temperature. This is called relative humidity. Humidity over 65% is an irritant and a trigger for people with asthma. There are reasons why hot, humid air may be problematic, such as that it is harder to breathe in and can activate sensory nerve fibers in the airways that stimulate coughing. These conditions are also the perfect breeding ground for asthma triggers, such as dust mites, mold, and pollen. Ozone levels are elevated, making the air stagnant and trapping pollutants such as car exhaust.

Part of the asthma action plan should be a way of dealing with humidity. Before going outdoors, check the local pollen and mold levels. When these factors are high, stay indoors in air conditioning as much as possible. Be sure also to take your controller medicine and always have your rescue inhaler on hand.

Using the Inhaler Properly

One of the major aspects of prevention and good care is using devices properly. Inhalers are probably the most misused of devices. If the goal is to avoid misuse, then one should do these things: checking the opening of the inhaler for debris such as crumbs, lint, and so forth from pockets; priming the inhaler if you have dropped it or if it has not been used in two weeks; shaking the inhaler to mix the medicine and propellant before use; exhaling before using so that your lungs have room for medicine; using a spacer to hold the medicine until you can breathe it in; waiting one minute between puffs; and rinsing your mouth after controller use, as not doing so can cause conditions such as thrush. Good techniques will ensure the person gets the needed medicine.

Wearing Medical Identification

Whether children or adults, people with asthma should have some type of device that identifies their medical condition. It can be a bracelet, necklace, or similar alert tag, which is worn at all times. If a severe attack occurs, and the person cannot explain the condition, the device will have the following information: list of major medical condition, allergies, and name and phone number of emergency contact. One device, Medic Alert (www.medicalert.org), provides a toll-free number that medical workers can call to find out this information.

Be Informed

Learn all you can about asthma. Know the condition, the medications, and the red lights. So many resources are available to learn about asthma. Refer to the Resource Section in the back of this book.

ASTHMA ACTION PLAN

For prevention and early intervention, everyone with asthma needs an asthma action plan. This plan will be coordinated with the person's healthcare provider and developed with the individual in mind. It should be written out and kept in a diary or notebook, which will have all the information collected in one place. The plan includes medicine, recognizing when the symptoms get worse, and what to do in an emergency. The following ideas are taken from the AAFA. There are other plan formats, but they generally include similar information.

Medicines

Page 1 should have the doctors' names and telephone numbers. It will have a graph of the name of the medication, how much, and how often it should be taken.

Recognizing When the Symptoms Change

The CDC sets these pages up with like a stoplight with green, yellow, and red. Below are the three stages:

- Green light. The person is feeling well, with no cough, wheezing, chest tightness, or trouble breathing at any time. The person can do all the things that he or she usually does without symptoms. When the person is tested with the peak flow meter, and the reading is more than 80% of the best peak flow, one must continue to take the long-term medication.

- Yellow light: Asthma is getting worse. Note if there are first signs of a cold or if the person has been exposed to a trigger. There is some coughing, wheezing, chest tightness, or trouble breathing. The person may wake up at night because of the asthma and cannot carry out usual activities. The peak flow meter is half to three-quarters of the best peak flow. Here one uses the quick-relief medicine and continue the long-term control medicine. If symptoms get better after an hour, keep checking them, but continue the long-term control medicine.

- Red light: Symptoms are bad. The person has a lot of trouble breathing, and the quick-relief medicine does not help. Nostrils are flared, and the person has trouble speaking. In children, the rib cage may be showing. The person cannot do normal activities. He or she was in the yellow zone for 24 hours but is not getting better. When the peak flow meter is tested, it is less than half of the best peak flow. Now is the time to add other medicines the doctor has prescribed and call the doctor. If the doctor cannot be reached, go to the hospital.

The plan includes what to do in an emergency. Parents need to work with health-care providers to develop emergency plans for what to do if the symptoms worsen. This may include more frequent use of a reliever medication and knowing when to call 911. Parents should not attempt to drive to the hospital because EMS staff evaluates asthma as soon as they arrive and can start treatment immediately; a dangerous complication could arise while driving to the hospital. The same advice goes for adults with asthma.

There are many electronic forms of the asthma plan that are available online. You can fill in the pertinent information and print out to include in the asthma diary.

It is very important for childcare providers to know about a child's asthma. If the child is in day care or preschool, giving them a written plan is a must. Likewise, such information should be provided to the school, which needs to share with teachers, school nurses, and staff.

Anyone with asthma needs an asthma action plan. The plan will give family, relatives, colleagues, and friends the necessary information regarding how to proceed in case of an asthma attack. And be sure to put it in a conspicuous place and inform people where to find it.

Tracking Asthma

An important part of managing asthma is learning the steps to take on a daily, weekly, monthly, or yearly basis. Doing this will require written tracking of symptoms. With your health-care professional, develop a system to track how often the flare-ups occur and how well medications are controlling the symptoms. Note any side effects, such as shaking, irritability, or trouble sleeping. Check lungs with a peak flow meter to see how well the lungs are working. Record how the symptoms affect daily activities such as work, play, sleep, or sports. Adjust medications when the symptoms get worse and know when to seek emergency care. Note the stoplight system of green, yellow, and red lights. Especially important is knowing the triggers and trying to avoid such things as colds, other respiratory infections, and pet dander.

Get involved in asthma education. Several websites and resources are available. Many of these are listed in this book. The CDC also has a website with resources for those dealing with asthma. https://www.cdc.gov/asthma/default.htm

MANAGING ASTHMA IN SCHOOLS

Pediatric asthma is affected by a range of factors, including exposure to triggers, changes in development and settings, and seasonality. Children spend over eight hours each weekday in school, and parents are not able to monitor the symptoms during those days. Thus, asthma treatment must be a collaborative effort among the student, family, and statewide agencies. School districts typically have limited resources to address asthma in the school setting. Thus, the management must involve a comprehensive approach across the home, school, and community.

Asthma is one of the leading causes of school absenteeism among children and adolescents in the United States. In a class of 30 children, about 3 are likely to have asthma. In low-income areas, the incidences may be higher. According to the CDC, the rate of asthma episodes is highest among Puerto Ricans, compared to all ethnic groups. The highest prevalence of asthma is highest among African American children, who also appear to die from asthma at a higher rate than people of other races or ethnicities. About 13.4% of African American children have asthma, compared to about 7.4% of white children with asthma.

Parents of children with chronic conditions may be surprised that many schools are not really equipped to deal with medical problems and emergencies. Much depends on the administration of the school to realize that they have the responsibility to address these issues. This is where parents may have to step in. Trained nurses are not always hired; some districts will have people with minimal training in charge of an area they may call a clinic. However, a school can become asthma friendly with a little attention.

Convince Administration of the Need

Using the statistics from the CDC, talk to the principal of the local school about the necessity for developing an asthma-friendly school. This is the place to start. Although it may seem more feasible to work with the district, the local school is the one that must deal with the children with the problem. Be aware that many schools—especially in low-income areas—may have many instances of asthma, but records are not kept for asthma incidences.

Lobby for an Asthma-Friendly School

Engage other parents of children who may suffer from asthma. You can do this by asking about it at parent meetings and having a general discussion about the problems others may be having. Most states require schools to have school improvement plans (SIPs). Make sure the health of children is included along with safe schools, discipline, reading, and math.

School Awareness

Make sure the school has a targeted list of those with the disorder. It should not be in the student's file but rather shared with the staff and other adults the child may come in contact with. This information is confidential and must be considered sensitive information. School must be aware of HIPAA laws.

With Permission, Examine the School Itself

Do not be afraid to ask questions. Some of the following questions will help you find out how well the school serves children with asthma: Are school buildings and grounds free of tobacco smoke at all times? Air from a designated place for smoking may waft into other rooms and halls. For children with a severe reaction to smoke, the smallest molecule of smoke can cause a reaction. Cigarette smoke can also cling to the clothes of people who are around it causing a reaction in some students. *Schools should be smoke-free zones.* Are school buses, vans, and trucks free of tobacco smoke? Are school events such as field trips and team games free of tobacco smoke? This should be a policy written in the school handbook.

Ask about Health Policies

Ask if the school allows students to carry and use their own asthma medicines. This could be a tricky problem. Students must understand that they cannot give or share or even show their medication to other students. But for some students, getting them to the health area may be a problem when time is of the essence. The student should understand where and whom to see if they have a problem. If the policy does not allow students to carry their own medicine, do the students have quick and easy access to the place where their medicines are stored?

Ask if there is a written plan for teachers and staff to follow if a student has an asthma attack. Consider how to handle emergencies such as a fire, tornado, severe weather, or a lockdown for safety concerns. What if a student forgets his or her medicine? Does the school have standing orders from health-care personnel for quick-relief medicines?

Student Asthma Action Plans on File

Make sure that all students with asthma have an asthma action plan from the student's doctor to help manage and prevent attacks.

Ideally, a school nurse should be in the building during all school hours. In any case, some responsible individual should be trained to help. That person should understand how to use medicines properly and encourage the student to be active in physical education, sports, recess, and field trips.

Education of Staff

Before teachers and staff can execute asthma plans and prevention, they themselves must be educated. This training should be done by health professionals who can talk about the conditions of asthma, medications, and prevention.

Options

Can students choose a physical activity that is different from others if medically necessary? Are medicines nearby before and after exercise? Also, if a different activity is chosen, it must not affect the grade in the physical education class.

Good Indoor Air Quality

Activists can check to make sure that the students are not subjected to allergens or irritants. School personnel must be aware that mold, dust mites, cockroaches, and strong odors from such things as aerosol sprays, bug spray, perfume, cleaners, or paint can be triggers for certain students.

Such a strong comprehensive program can ensure parents that their children are getting the care they need, and students can live healthy happy lives. Asthma cannot be cured, but it can be controlled. The school can then concentrate on its mission of teaching. Many resources are available to assist families and school staff. Refer to the section of resources in the back of this book.

Community and Prevention

The community can play a strong role in prevention and care of people with asthma. For example, in the state of Rhode Island, there is an evidence-based program whose goals are to reduce asthma-related emergency department visits and enhance home-based environmental hazards. Called the HARP program (Home Asthma Response Plan), the program provides guidelines-based asthma education to caregivers of children with asthma in the home setting conducted by a certified asthma educator. The educators show the family how to deal with and control triggers in the home. Families in the program received three home visits to ensure that strategies are understood, and there are opportunities for problem-solving if barriers arise. In addition, the program helps with the development of the asthma action plan. Results have shown this program is effective in reducing ER visits and hospitalizations.

CONCLUSION

Remember that asthma cannot be cured, but it can be controlled. This chapter has focused on prevention and early detection. We have examined such topics as practicing good personal care, vaccines, lifestyle changes, and asthma action plans. Because children spend so much time in school, we have focused on how the school can become asthma-friendly. The general communities and the health-care community also have roles to play. Several overall comprehensive prevention plans are available. The problem is that many do not realize that help is available and do not take the initiative to combat ER visits through education. There are several resources in the back of the book listing the agencies and groups that are ready to help.

9

Issues and Controversies

In recent years, there has been an explosion of information about the causes and treatments of asthma. Understanding of the pathogenesis and therapy has undoubtedly improved over the last few years. However, although the knowledge of asthma has increased, so have morbidity and mortality. No general agreement exists on the reasons for such an increase. That problem is the emphasis of this chapter. One of the areas of disagreement is the genetic causes of the condition. Although much research is available in this area, scientists disagree on significant findings. Several controversies exist in the clinical management of the disease, such as the best maintenance therapy, the role of beta-agonists, the role of inflammation, functions of nebulized beta-agonists, and, lastly, the role of immunotherapy. We will explore the status of emerging and experimental therapies in chapter 10, "Current Research and Future Directions." With the advent of the worldwide pandemic of COVID-19 in 2020, questions about the relationship between asthma and COVID-19 and other viruses is a current and controversial subject for consideration.

THE GENETICS OF ASTHMA

People have noted for many years that asthma and other similar disorders run in families. However, the connection appears to be elusive and not well understood. During recent decades, research into genetic causes has exploded. The researchers have found that allergy and asthma complexes do not conform to Mendelian inheritance's simple pattern, such as Huntington disease or sickle-cell disease.

A single gene with two alleles, one from each parent, controls these traits. One of the alleles may be dominant over the other and appear as characteristics. Like many different conditions, such as hypertension (high blood pressure), diabetes, or psychotic conditions, asthma is a complex genetic disorder. The search to determine candidate genes and the specific places on the genes, called loci, is very demanding and challenging.

Until recently, such research was purely theoretical. However, the revolution in molecular genetics has made it possible to locate specific DNA sequences that constitute the genetic risk factors for developing allergies and asthma. Several things are known about the genetic connection.

Scientists know that asthma and allergies have a familial connection. This connection can be due to the individuals sharing the same environment as well as shared genes. The study of twins has given great insight into this principle. Identical twins are monozygotic, meaning they arose from one fertilized egg divided into two individuals sharing the same genetic makeup. Fraternal twins occur from two fertilized eggs and have the same genetic makeup only to the same extent as any other sibling. Studies of twins can help determine the contribution of shared environment and genetic makeup. Also, identical twins raised apart contribute to this study.

In twin studies, Simon Thomsen (2015b) found that asthma is highly heritable, with genetic factors accounting for 70% of the variation in susceptibility. However, only about 35% accounted for age at onset and around 25% in variation of the disease's severity. According to the author, twin studies have substantiated the hygiene hypothesis, fetal origins hypothesis, autoimmune disease, and metabolic syndrome. Future twin studies should examine more advanced molecular methods within epigenetics and microbiome analysis.

Tracing the prevalence of genetic factors in a family also has enlightened researchers. Segregation analysis examines the transmission of the trait to see how it conforms to genetic and environmental patterns. There are numerous studies of the design of inheritance of asthma, rhinitis, allergic dermatitis, and IgE serum levels. These studies have shown that the conditions are at least partly due to shared genes. Some authors have concluded that the genetic contribution is more important than environmental factors. This point of view is controversial.

A second known item is that both asthma and allergy inheritance are polygenic, meaning several genes are involved. These conditions have a non-Mendelian pattern of inheritance that is characteristic of complex genetic disorders. Another feature of complex genetic diseases is genetic heterogeneity or different combinations of gene variants contributing to the condition's appearance in other families.

Evidence exists that the inheritance of these disorders is end-organ specific. This idea means that the conditions locate in a particular place, such as the airways, nose, or skin. Although an exaggerated IgE response may underlie the disease, separate genes within the family may show a different allergic reaction type.

Specific areas of the human genome harbor the susceptibility for allergy and asthma. In 1989, Cookson and a team first reported they had identified a locus containing a gene related to atopic dermatitis on chromosome 11q.

Several methods have found specific genes that contribute to asthma and allergy. An older method is called classic linkage in multigenerational families. More recently, the sib-pair method detects excessive pairing of parental alleles. These methods, along with some others, have identified several loci involved in the pathogenesis of asthma. The problem arises when other investigators are not able to reproduce these results.

Thomsen (2015b) wrote a comprehensive review of research at the time. The team expressed the idea that the risk of disease depends on the degree of genetic relatedness. These factors are both genetic and environmental and appear to involve the interaction of several genes with environmental factors.

These studies take a tremendous amount of time and involve many genetic centers at universities or private facilities. Currently, Moffatt et al. (2010) conducted the largest and most comprehensive study by a consortium of 100 centers worldwide. The team studied the genotypes of 10,365 persons with asthma and compared the associates to 16,110 unaffected persons. The extensive study identified the following genes on chromosomes associated with asthma: chromosomes 2 (*IL1RL1/IL18R1*), 6 (*HLA-DQ*), 9 (*IL33*), 15 (*SMAD3*), 17 (*ORMDL3/GSDMB*), and 22 (*IL2RB*). Specifically, the ORMDL13 gene was associated with childhood-onset asthma; the HLA-DQ gene was related to later-onset asthma.

Many questions exist about the genetic relationship. For example, are there separate genetic contributions for increased IgE levels? What linkages are due to the presence of specific other genes or gene complexes? And importantly, do we have the current knowledge and technology to discover novel genes? These searches are very costly. Will companies invest in gene discovery? And most of all, if we identify a gene, are there preventive or therapeutic procedures to help those persons with asthma?

This chapter has considered questions and controversies relating to genetics. Chapter 10 will go a step further to look at the future of molecular genetics and how it will integrate into an area called personalized medicine.

CONTROVERSIES SURROUNDING ASTHMA TREATMENTS

Asthma is a reversible disorder caused by smooth muscle contractions of the bronchial tubes; however, patients with severe conditions have extensive inflammatory changes of the airways, including plugs of mucous, extensive sloughing of the epithelial lining, and extensive inflammation of the cells of the mucosa and submucosa. The use of certain medicines has been recommended and appears to help, at least for a while. Several researchers are now questioning if these treatments might contribute to airway inflammation.

Inhaled Steroids

Numerous studies have shown that inhaled steroids can control chronic asthma symptoms; however, the side effects may be a potential problem. The toxic reaction varies with the total dose, the dosing schedule, use of a spacer, mouth rinsing, and how the effect is measured. Adverse effects are in two categories: topical and systemic.

Topical side effects can be dealt with if used correctly and in regular doses. However, some people develop a sore mouth or throat, a hoarse or croaky voice (called dysphonia), and a cough. Oral thrush or candidiasis is a fungal infection that causes white patches, redness, or soreness in the mouth. Some individuals develop nosebleeds. The person can usually control these side effects with slow inhalation, a spacer device, and gargling.

Systemic side effects are even more concerning. The hypothalamic-pituitary-adrenal (HPA) axis is a complex set of interactions among three areas: the hypothalamus, located deep in the brain; the pituitary gland, also in the brain, which is considered the master control of other glands; and the adrenal glands, located on top of the kidneys. The use of inhaled steroids can affect the HPA, causing adverse effects on bone metabolism and eventually osteoporosis, slowing growth in children and adolescents, cataracts, bruising, dermal thinning, and psychological changes. Although the response may vary among individuals, studies have shown that an excess of 800μg/day in adults and 400μg/day in children can suppress the HPA. Inhaled corticosteroids as low as 400μg/day have been associated with the development of osteoporosis.

The Cromes

Two drugs, cromolyn sodium (CS) and nedocromil sodium (NS), are alternated initial controlled therapies for mild asthma in national and international guidelines. Although inhaled glucocorticosteroids are preferred, these two have a lower incidence of side effects.

Cromolyn Sodium

Several studies have documented that CS prevents asthma symptoms against allergens, cold air, SO_2, and exercise. It does appear to be less effective against methacholine and histamine. Several studies have proposed that the CS has an effect on nonspecific bronchial hyperactivity. It seems to be most effective when administered as a preventative. The drug was first available in the 1970s, but as of 9/2020 availability varies from country to country due to the change of propellants used in metered-dose inhalers. Although none of these devices are sold in the United States, inhalers containing hydrofluroalkane (HFA) are available in the United Kingdom and a Spinhaler in Australia.

Nedocromil Sodium

Nedocromil sodium (NS) was approved in the United States in 1993 for use in metered-dose inhalers (MDIs.) NS is structurally different from CS but has a similar pharmacologic mechanism of action. In the United States, neither CS nor NS is available in HFA-containing MDIs, and no formulation of NS is marketed for asthma. Only cromolyn (10mg. mL) solutions for nebulization are available; dry powder inhaled drugs are available in other countries. Although they represent an alternative therapy, the two remain controversial but have no clear advantage over inhaled steroids and cost more.

Do Beta-Agonists Increase Deaths?

Beta-adrenergic drugs or agonists are the most potent bronchodilators approved for clinical use for asthma. However, controversy does surround the use of β-agonists in the increasing mortality rate. Researchers in one study hypothesize that such bronchodilators worsen asthma and contribute to morbidity and mortality. As early as 1983, Grant and a group of researchers in New Zealand suggested that inhaled β-agonists increase the risk of death in severe asthma. Spitzer et al. (1992), using health insurance data from Saskatchewan with 12,301 patients, found an increased risk of death with asthma, an odds ratio of 5.4 per canister of fenoterol and 2.44 per canister of albuterol.

Nwaru et al. (2020) investigated the overuse of SABA by linking data from Swedish national registries. They found that one-third of asthma patients in Sweden collected three or more SABA canisters annually, and this overuse was associated with increased risks of exacerbation and asthma mortality.

Although the exact contribution of β-agonists to increased mortality trends remains unknown, there is sufficient reason for concern. β-agonists are a critical part of the acute emergency management of bronchial asthma. However, they probably should be avoided in long-term care maintenance.

Role of Inflammation

The role of inflammation in asthma is a subject of controversy. Also, the importance of inflammation in a subset of people who develop sudden decomposition is poorly understood. Numerous retrospective studies have examined the relationship between asthma and death. They classified deaths as type 1 with a slow-onset or type 2 with a sudden onset.

Type 1 onset is the result of several interacting factors. These include severe asthma requiring ER visits and mechanical ventilation. Certain socioeconomic factors, psychological features, race, and culture appear to interfere with compliance or medical care access. The person might have had improper pulmonary testing or inadequate treatment with inhaled or systemic anti-inflammatory procedures. In these cases, someone has probably not taken the symptoms seriously.

Several researchers have investigated circumstances when patients die suddenly and unexpectedly of Type 2 asthma. Wasserfallen et al. (1995) found three patterns in 34 patients who required intubation and mechanical ventilation. These patterns were: rapid or less than 3 hours; gradual of 9.2 days, plus or minus 7.7 days; and acute after an unstable attack of 4.2 days, plus or minus 3.6 days. The sudden type was more frequent in young men with excess CO_2 in the bloodstream. The authors suggested that bronchospasm was the primary cause in this group. In another study of 81 patients who had fewer than 3 lapsed hours from attack to mechanical intubation, Kallenbach et al. (1993) found a higher mortality rate. Sur et al. (1993) studied histological differences and found in the sudden-onset group that neutrophils exceeded eosinophils in the airway submucosa, indicating that the immunology of sudden onset is distinct from slow-onset asthma.

The studies above have established basic questions about the role of inflammation. At the 2015 Aspen Lung Conference, participants questioned the paradigm that airway inflammation is at the center of asthma pathogenesis. The presenters believed that inflammation could no longer explain critical elements of our current knowledge about the disease. The conference came to two conclusions: (1) epidemiological, genetic, epigenetic, experimental, and clinical evidence indicate that airways epithelium and airway smooth muscles are potential sites for the primary derangement in the different kinds of asthmas; and (2) to improve the lives of patients with severe or difficult-to-treat asthma, renewed studies for identifying molecular markers such as genetic, genomic, and epigenetic to classify patients into specific types are essential. Chapter 10 will discuss these efforts in detail.

WHAT IS THE ROLE OF EMERGENCY MANAGEMENT?

For people with severe or acute asthma, the best way to administer help is a subject of disagreement. There is controversy over the best way to administer β-agonists and whether the use of aminophylline is appropriate.

Should patients use nebulized continuous or intermittent β-agonists? Several studies found comparable results in emergency management for bronchodilation with both an MDI and a nebulizer. However, patients with acute airflow may need higher dosages of the aerosol. Several studies have found that, rather than intermittent administration, β-agonists may be useful when given in continuous intervals. Hospital standard therapy for acutely ill patients involves giving the β-agonist at 20- to 30-minute intervals. People with acute airflow may be candidates for continuous treatment with nebulized bronchodilators while waiting for anti-inflammatory therapy. Extensive experience with children suggests this approach is safe, although further studies may be essential for adults with underlying coronary disease. In current research, Kulalert et al. (2020) found that continuous SABA nebulization was more efficient in treating children with severe asthma exacerbation; adults were not included in this study.

Aminophylline

Aminophylline is a compound of the bronchodilator theophylline with ethylenediamine in a 2:1 ratio. The use of aminophylline in the treatment of acute, severe asthma is controversial. For example, Littenberg (1988) did a meta-analysis of 13 controlled studies and found no overall benefit of using aminophylline: three studies favored administering the drug; three favored a control regimen consisting of albuterol, epinephrine, or other bronchodilators; and seven found no difference. The current consensus is that patients with acute asthma, who require hospitalization and may not respond to other treatments, receive the medication.

Role of Immunotherapy

Immunotherapy is a treatment that uses certain parts of a person's immune system to fight a disease or disorder. It works by stimulating or boosting your immune system's natural defenses so that it can fight off the conditions causing the disease. Researchers developed the idea of using immunotherapy to treat allergic disorders in the early 1900s; however, using it to treat asthma is controversial due to several factors. Generally, the target of immunotherapy is for the type of asthma related to allergies. The pathogenesis of the role of asthma triggers, both allergic and nonallergenic, is not well defined. Also, immunotherapy is not standardized in its potency, preparation methods of administration, and duration.

Graft and Valentine (1993) analyzed 100 controlled studies of immunotherapy to treat asthma, some of which were double-blinded. They found evidence to support the use of dust mite extract, pollen extract, and dog and cat dander extract for cases triggered by these specific allergens. Few studies of mold have been done, and most of these were done in Europe. The treatments are controversial because not all studies of immunotherapy have shown benefit. Some showed decreases in responsiveness after long-term use.

Since this study, research on immunotherapy has continued, and chapter 10 will consider several other reviews and the potential for the future of immunotherapy. However, it is used for those who cannot control asthma by avoiding standard asthma medications. Conditions for the use of immunotherapy are as follows: (1) triggers correlate with a specific situation; (2) avoidance is not possible; (3) patient cannot tolerate asthma medicines because of toxicity or adverse events; (4) the person's occupation such as veterinarians or farm workers prohibits avoidance; (5) seasonal rhinitis occurs with seasonal asthma; and (6) risks and benefits are discussed with the patient. Immunotherapy can be life-threatening. Some patients may have severe reactions to allergy shots.

THE HYGIENE HYPOTHESIS: PROS AND CONS

This idea or theory suggests a child's environment can be too clean, which hampers the immune system's development. In the late 1980s, David P. Strachan, a British professor of epidemiology, published an article in the *British Medical Journal*. He followed 17,000 children born in 1958 and found that children in larger households had fewer hay fever cases because they were exposed to germs by the older siblings. Other researchers investigated the idea. In the late 1990s, Dr. Erika von Mutius studied the rates of allergies and asthma in East Germany and West Germany, unified in 1999.

She found that children in the polluted areas of East Germany, which were generally dirtier and less healthful, had fewer cases than children in the West. Additional research has found that children in developing areas of the world were much less likely to have asthma and allergies than children in the developed world. Naturally, these findings were controversial and caused a stir among the health community.

Pro Arguments for the Hygiene Hypothesis

Babies inside the uterus are protected by the mother's antibodies and thus have a fragile immune system. When they are born, the immune system must start working on its own. For this system to work correctly, the child must be exposed to organisms to build immunity. Think of the immune system as a bodybuilder. The person trains the muscles by lifting heavier and more massive objects; if the muscles are not trained, they will be unfit and unable to raise a heavy object. So it is with the immune system. To fight off infection, the person must train the immune system by fighting off contaminants encountered in everyday life.

Understanding how the immune system evolves and works is essential to this theory. Mutius hypothesized that there are two types of biological defenses: first, one system does not fight off infection; the other system overcompensates and creates an allergic reaction to harmless substances like pollen.

The Science behind the Theory

Before birth, the fetal immune system is set to suppress it from rejecting maternal tissue. Epidemiologic studies demonstrate that allergic diseases and asthma occur with the incidence of low levels of an endotoxin called a bacterial lipopolysaccharide (LPS) in the home. LPS stimulates and educates the immune system by triggering a molecular switch called TLR4, located on specific immune system cells. The FDA's Inflammatory Mechanisms Section of the Laboratory of Immunobiochemistry has looked at the relationship between respiratory viruses, especially respiratory syncytial virus (RSV), and allergic diseases and asthma. They have found the following relationship: RSV is often the first pathogen encountered by infants; RSV pneumonia puts babies at a higher risk for childhood asthma; and RSV carries a molecule on the surface called the F protein, which flips the same immune system switch (TLR4) as do bacterial endotoxins. The FDA admits that studying the effect of RSV on T cells in the laboratory is difficult. They concluded from the study that a newborn's immune system must be educated to function correctly during a person's life. The critical element appears to be TLR4 on the T cells. The laboratory is continuing its research on TLR and RSV and how they contribute to the hygiene effect.

Adding to the controversy in 1997, some people began to question if there is a correlation between the hygiene hypothesis and vaccinations. With the number of vaccinations going up, so did the number of children with allergies and other immune-related problems. The question developed is depriving the immune system of infections using vaccines causing the system to attack itself. This idea had been disproven in three studies reviewed by Herbarth et al. (2015). These studies showed that vaccines did not correlate with children developing allergies and ailments later in life. Vaccination may help prevent asthma and other health problems in addition to the diseases they targeted.

Con Arguments against the Hygiene Hypothesis

Several researchers have expressed concern about hygiene attitudes and think that people should not use the term hygiene. They believe that this theory undermines attitudes toward real hygiene, and the misnaming could contribute to the spread of infectious disease. They question the fundamental premise that the rapid rise in childhood allergies is due to the lack of exposure to childhood infections, smaller family sizes, and higher home and personal hygiene standards. Much publicity has promoted the link between being too clean and the development of asthma. However, to link the two is incorrect.

The researchers explained that the exposure that is needed is not to infections but beneficial microbes. In our bodies is a large body of microorganisms called the microbiome. These organisms function to keep the immune system from overreacting to harmless stimuli, such as pollen or foods.

In 2003, Dr. Graham Rook of University College, London, proposed an alternative hypothesis. He said that during human evolution, microbes have evolved into an essential part of our immune system. These are beneficial microbes that do not cause infection but are acquired by exposure to humans or animals from our natural environment. He named this the "old friends hypothesis." Early exposure to a range of friendly pathogens, not infectious pathogens, is necessary to train the immune system. He emphasized that the organisms we evolved to acquire are our mothers and organisms' microbiota from the natural environment. The unique biome starts before we are born as maternal microbes colonize in the human gut and then pass through the birth canal and are breastfed. Young children amass these from contact with every family member and while playing outside in the dirt, getting licked by dogs, and sharing toys with friends. Continuing to call it the hygiene hypothesis is wrong.

As Rook was developing his theory, scientists found regulatory T cells, which challenge the immune responses. He proposed that exposure to nonpathogenic microbes activates various immune processes, including T cells, to regulate the immune system properly. The researcher likens the immune system to a computer to software, but the design needs data in the form of a diverse set to microbes to train it properly. He also has linked the Caesarian section to the increased risk of allergy and asthma. Owning a pet or growing up on a farm protects, but antibiotic use, which kills off both good and bad microbes, has been linked to asthma.

Sally Bloomfield, from the London School of Hygiene and Tropical Medicine, believes that there is little to no evidence that the adverse effects resulting from personal or household hygiene or cleanliness. But she is concerned that the hygiene hypothesis misnomer is confusing the public and making them distrustful of health practices.

Bloomfield and her colleagues are calling for change. She emphasized that we are still a long way from knowing the beneficial microbes. We know that acceptable hygiene practices, such as handwashing, food hygiene, and respiratory hygiene, prevent harmful microbes. We must tackle antibiotic resistance and take charge of our health.

Striking a balance is essential. The conflict between cleanliness and exposure can leave parents confused. Of course, many microbes can make people sick such as the respiratory syncytial virus (RSV), *E. coli, salmonella*, and so on. People need to be aware of where these bacteria are and take care to avoid them. But the role of good bacteria is not well understood by the general public, which is clear from the fact that many think that taking antibiotics for every small problem is the answer. Of course, cleaning the house is very important. The CDC recommends regular cleaning and disinfecting certain areas of the house, especially when surfaces might have contact with feces or meat or with someone who is ill.

The balancing act should help one understand when bacteria and viruses may cause illness, and when cleaning is beneficial. Children should be encouraged to play outside even if they get dirty. However, creating a healthy lifestyle is part of the balancing act.

ASTHMA, COVID-19, AND OTHER VIRUSES

In 2020, an illness called COVID-19 started spreading, causing a worldwide pandemic. This section is included because of the virus's current unknown longevity and its possible relationship to future viruses.

Coronaviruses are a group of viruses. They are classified as RNA viruses, which have ribonucleic (RNA) as genetic material. RNA nucleic acid is usually single-stranded compared to deoxyribonucleic acid (DNA), which is double-stranded. RNA viruses cause the common cold, influenza, SARS, MERS, Dengue fever, hepatitis C, West Nile fever, Ebola, rabies, polio, and measles.

Coronaviruses cause respiratory tract infections ranging from mild to lethal; a specific virus, SARS-CoV-2, causes COVID-19. The first case was identified in Wuhan, China, in December 2019. According to the CDC, COVID-19 symptoms include fever, chills, cough, shortness of breath or trouble breathing, tiredness, muscle aches, body aches, headache, loss of smell and taste, and sore throat.

People with asthma are concerned about telling the difference between asthma, COVID-19, flu, common cold, or seasonal allergies. Any respiratory condition can worsen asthma, but if you have a fever or cough, contact the doctor. Asthma is on some lists of conditions that put people at high risk; other lists do not. It concerns asthmatic patients who already experience respiratory symptoms. The CDC says that although there is no evidence that people with asthma are more likely to contract the disease. The agency does warn that patients with moderate-to-severe who contract COVID-19 are at a higher risk of severe complications, including asthma attacks, pneumonia, and acute respiratory distress.

COVID-19 and other viruses are a controversial concern, especially with figures relating to the mortality of patients. Wang et al. (2021) did a systematic review and meta-analysis of the relationship between asthma and the increase in patients' mortality with COVID-19. The study found a limited number of studies. They count that the evidence suggests that asthma as comorbidity may not significantly prolong the hospital stay or risk for ICU transfer. They did find that comorbidities such as hypertension, diabetes, COPD, malignancy, obesity, immunosuppression, and renal disease increase the risk of mortality in patients with COVID-19. However, the role of asthma in influencing related outcomes is unclear, according to the authors. Although this study did have many limitations, it was the first meta-analysis showing asthma's influence on the results of COVID-19 patients. Thus, preliminary data indicate that asthma as comorbidity may not increase the mortality of COVID-19, but data of hospitalization, duration, and ICU admission is still limited.

CONCLUSION

Medical care and lifestyle are always controversial subjects, and the best asthma strategies are specific, no exceptions. Recent information about the causes and treatment of asthma has exploded. Understanding of the pathogenesis and therapy has undoubtedly improved over the last few years. However, although the knowledge and recent information about the causes and treatment have exploded during the past decade, there will always be arguments about what is best and what we should do. No general agreement exists on the reasons for such an increase. This chapter has considered several controversial topics. Research into genetics and personalized medicine for asthma have emerged in the last few decades; however, there are still many questions and no real definitive answers. Clinical treatments have several controversies and problems. For example, what is the best maintenance therapy, what is the role of beta-agonists, where does inflammation fit in, what are the best strategies for functions of nebulized beta-agonists, and lastly, is immunotherapy effective and useful? We looked in detail at the hygiene hypothesis, which most researchers now think is a misnomer and should be called the "old friends hypothesis." A section on COVID-19 is included because of its controversial relationship to asthma. As we consider the future of asthma in chapter 10, we will most certainly encounter treatments that will be controversies in the future.

10

Current Research and Future Directions

Look up the word "asthma" in any search engine, and you will find more than 76 million entries. These searches illustrate that people are looking for help now but also looking to the future. Hankin et al. (2013) still remind us that severe and uncontrolled asthma is prevalent; they show the gap between medicine offers and expectations. There are more than 150,000 articles in peer-reviewed journals, with nearly 6% reporting the results of randomized control trials. However, although many therapeutic trials exist, routine options to treat asthma remain relatively narrow and strongly dominated by steroids.

Let us imagine the future of asthma. If we are realistic, we must combine the outlooks of patients and their families, clinicians working with patients, basic and clinical researchers, and the industry. This chapter will include all these points of view. We will discuss the future of disease modifiers, types of immunotherapy, behavior modification, genetics, drug delivery, improving existing drugs through nanotechnology, and the all-important topic of personalized medicine.

DISEASE MODIFIERS

Prediction about the onset of asthma is of great interest. When and where attacks will occur are becoming elusive topics. Today, many researchers worldwide seek to define and locate strategies for changing or modifying the disease. Disease modifiers include challenging and evolving risks. Many of the treatment plans are lacking in this area. The hope relies on the intervention's ability to affect the disease's natural history, but showing prevention efficacy is quite tricky. Immunotherapy has had some success in stopping the disease's progress but does not indicate a reduced risk of development. Inhaled corticosteroids certainly do not reduce risk. Hence, scientists are investigating other strategies to counter the effect.

Bronchial Thermoplasty

Thermoplasty, as the name implies, uses heat to treat airways. Approved by the FDA in 2010 as a strategy to reduce airway stiffness and excessive narrowing, scientists found that a limited number of patients show improvement using bronchial thermoplasty (Dombret et al., 2014). Researchers at Cleveland Clinic's Respiratory Institute use the strategy as part of comprehensive management and treatment for asthma and, at present, remains the only approved non-pharmacologic device. As an outpatient procedure, technicians insert a catheter into the bronchial tubes to deliver precisely controlled thermal energy to the airways. Because asthma leads to increased airway smooth muscle constricting breathing, the modality reduces ASM thickness and improves airflow's airflow ability. According to the Cleveland Clinic, patients have demonstrated significant improvement and reduced the number of flare-ups.

The treatment includes three separate bronchoscopic procedures about three weeks apart: one for each lower lobe and another for the upper lobe. The patient is sedated, and a thin, flexible tube is inserted through the patient's nose or mouth into the lungs. The candidate must be between the ages of 18 and 65 and have a history of severe asthma that is not controlled by steroids.

Yale Center for Asthma and Airway Disease has also had success with the procedure. Bronchial thermoplasty is delivered by the Alair® System using thermal energy to reduce the muscle associated with airway constriction. Clinical studies have shown sustained improvements in asthma control up to a year following the treatment, along with fewer severe asthma attacks, visits to the ER, and fewer lost days from work or school.

A downside is the increase in the frequency and worsening of respiratory symptoms immediately following the procedure. The events may occur within one to seven days. Hospitalization afterward may be recommended.

Epigenetic Modifications

Epigenetic modifications are the next important step in reducing risk. These changes involve DNA. They are persistent and heritable and regulate the expression of genes, but they are not the gene itself. Examples include DNA methylation, histone modifications, and microRNA regulation. The modification involves an understanding of which epigenetic changes are responsible for asthma, the implications for onset and maintenance of the disease, and the risks of treatment. Studies of microRNA, especially the use of antagomirs, a class of chemically engineered molecules that prevent other molecules from binding to the desired site on an mRNA molecule, also fit into risk reduction. (See section on epigenetic research in this chapter.)

TYPES OF IMMUNOTHERAPIES

The chronic inflammatory condition of asthma involves numerous cells and cellular elements that play a role. For over 100 years, various forms of subcutaneous immunotherapy with allergen extracts have been in use. Jutel et al. (2015) codified an international consensus on allergy immuno-therapy (AIT). They concluded that despite numerous clinical trials and meta-analyses showing AIT's effectiveness, it remains underused, and estimates are that less than 10% of patients with allergic rhinitis worldwide have been treated with AIT. The consensus is that AIT is the only treat-ment that can change the allergic disease course by preventing asthma and new allergens. The international community of allergy specialists recog-nizes the need to develop comprehensive guidelines.

Sublingual Immunotherapy (SLIT)

As of 2020, SLIT is a safe, effective treatment for allergic rhinitis. It has significant usage in European countries but limited clinical use in the United States. The FDA has approved three SLIT tablets for allergic rhini-tis and allergic rhinoconjunctivitis concerning pollen: Grastek® and Oralair® for grass pollen and Ragwitek™ for ragweed pollen. Physicians can prescribe SLIT off-label for other conditions, but the barriers of additional formulations, standard dose, dosing schedule, and cost/insurance cover-age remain. Researchers are exploring SLIT use for allergic asthma, food allergies, atopic dermatitis, and other diseases. At present, the future of SLIT is unknown.

AIT with Recombinant Allergens

Allergic immunotherapy (AIT) is based on allergen-specific forms of intervention. It requires identification of the disease-causing allergens before creating the prescription for the correct AIT. Zhernov et al. (2019) reviewed the state of this strategy's art and found it cost-effective and the only disease-modifying treatment for allergy; its limitations are the low quality of natural allergen extracts. AIT is based on recombinant and synthetic allergen derivations, which induce allergen-specific blockers of IgE. It is clinically effective and can overcome the limitations of allergen extracts. On the horizon are vaccination and tolerance induction strategies. According to Zhernov, lack of resources is a significant problem for developing new AIT molecular strategies. These barriers hinder AIT allergy prevention from transitioning from the bench to the clinic.

Immunotherapy with Peptides

Klein et al. (2019) published an article in a French journal of mouse model studies showing that hypoallergenic peptides from allergens can prevent airway hyperresponsiveness, decrease Th2 response, and decrease allergen-specific IgE. Some of the peptides' mechanisms are unknown, but their effectiveness with low doses of allergens makes peptide immunotherapy a promising novel approach to inflammatory responses.

Toll-Like Receptors (TLRs) against Inflammation

These receptors play a vital role in the innate immune system. Researchers have TLRs to up-regulate the Th1 responses and down-regulate the Th2 responses in mouse models of allergic or chronic asthma. Leaker et al. (2019) examined the efficacy and safety of the TRL7 agonist AZD8848, which was developed as an antedrug, a substance given before treatment. They found that in patients with allergic asthma, TLR7 agonists reduced allergen responsiveness by stimulating Type 1 interferon responses to down-regulate the dominant Th2 responses.

Monoclonal Antibodies (MABs)

Monoclonal antibodies (MABs) are a type of laboratory-made protein that can bind to substances of one kind—hence the name "monoclonal."

MABs have been developed to target eosinophilic inflammation in Type 2 asthma. The FDA has approved Omalizumab (anti-IgE) (Xolair®) for the treatment of severe allergic asthma. Mepolizumab (anti-IL-5) reduces exacerbation in patients with severe eosinophilic asthma. Other MABs are in development to target allergic and eosinophilic inflammation.

Edris et al. (2019) performed a meta-analysis of 30 trials and the effects of these biologics that target the IL-5, IL-13, IL-4, I-9, Il-2, and TSLP receptors. They found the MABs such as mepolizumab (NUCALA ®), reslizumab, and benralizumab reduce severe persistent eosinophilic asthma in published trials.

Autoantibodies

An autoantibody is a protein produced by the immune system directed against one or more of the person's proteins. Many autoimmune diseases, such as lupus, are caused by autoantibodies. Researchers have attempted to generate autoantibody responses to the cytokines implicated in asthma. These therapies seek to modify the Th2 immune response, which is involved with many forms of asthma.

BEHAVIOR MODIFICATION

Behavior modification (B-Mod) is a treatment approach that targets changing behaviors. It replaces undesirable behaviors with more desirable ones using operant conditioning principles, ideas developed by psychologist B. F. Skinner. Working with individuals or families, a trained specialist will focus on the behavior, emphasizing current environmental events. There will be a detailed description of the targeted problems, and the person will help work out a plan to change these behaviors. It is often used with asthma patients and their families to develop a workable asthma plan.

Of course, the best strategy for the prevention of asthma is avoiding asthma onset. To prevent this, people must identify those at risk, especially newborns and children, and then modify risky behaviors.

Predictive Index

Chang et al. (2013) developed an Modified Asthma Predictive Index (mAPI) that measured sensitivity, specificity, positive likelihood reaction, negative likelihood ratio, and post-test probabilities of asthma in unselected and high-risk populations from ages 6 to 11. In a high-risk cohort, a positive mAPI is correlated with the probability of future asthma. Bisgaard et al. (2012) showed that measuring airway obstruction very early in life is also appropriate as it suggests inheritance of bronchial airway issues far earlier than immune system maturation. The study found that children developing asthma by age seven had a lung function deficit and increased bronchial responsiveness as neonates. These children did not have exposure to the condition that develops T-helper cell responses early in life. This study is in line with the hygiene hypothesis of the broad diversity of exposure to specific antigens to build the immune system. Other studies discuss the role of diet, antibiotics, restricting cesarean delivery, avoiding maternal and environmental smoke exposure, promoting breastfeeding, and decreasing a hyper-hygienic environment.

ROLE OF THE HYGIENE HYPOTHESIS

The question here about the hygiene hypothesis is how much exposure and what is a critical number of microbial exposure. Schuijs et al. (2015) found a relationship to the A20 protein, a tumor necrosis factor-A-induced protein 3. A20 regulates the interactions between dendritic cells and the airway epithelium. An A20 single-nucleotide polymorphism increases the risk of asthma and allergy in children who grew up on farms, and A20 modulations affect asthma development, according to Schuss et al. (2015).

Modern Psychological Insight

Chanez and Humbert (2011) did a thought-provoking study (in French) entitled, "When patients and caregivers are both in trouble, can we assume the relationship is difficult?" (translation). The authors proposed that especially with difficult-to-treat cases, the age of the Internet has caused a new relationship between patients and physicians. Doctor consultations are more complex and tense as "expert" patients and caregivers have become more anxious, skeptical, and prone to self-diagnose. Several doctors, interested in their patients' adherence, placed microchips in medical devices without their patients' consent or knowledge. Are such practices ethical? Also, what is the role of social networks? Should patients who are "friends" with their doctors follow them on Twitter? The French Medical Association ruled against this in 2011, warning practitioners against patients and doctors on the Internet. Is virtual closeness valuable? What about online support groups? Would asthma be better controlled? And who could control that? The French researchers asked these questions in this study but did not have the answers.

FUTURE OF ASTHMA GENETICS

Genetics, with all its research and glitz, poses a significant problem for asthma researchers. Indeed, understanding natural history and pathogenesis has developed, but this effort has not translated into new or modifiable treatments. Many genes regulate asthma, and each of these contributes in a subtle way to diseases. Most known genes may increase the risk by about a factor of 1.2 or less. Geneticists have shown that asthma does not vary in the phenotype or manifestation but is very heterogeneous genetically.

Next-Generation Sequencing and Genomic Analysis

The Human Genome Project used a relatively small number of genomes to sequence the 21,000 genes. Efforts are going forward to create a reference genome that will analyze human genes. The 1000 Genomes Project (2012) was initiated to sequence many people's genomes and provide a comprehensive genetic variation resource. The challenge lies in interpreting such a large quantity of data and implementing it into clinical practice and counseling with families.

Some strategies target the clinical characteristics of asthma. Atopy is probably the first phenotypic trait to target for personalized treatment. Atopy refers to the genetic tendency to develop allergic diseases such as rhinitis, asthma, and eczema. Avoidance and immunotherapy are two cornerstones of the management, and adding a rescue drug such as omalizumab may still be insufficient. New outlooks on the anti-IgE blockade may improve IgE binding. Gauvreau et al. (2014) found that the optimal frequency of administration of quilizumab may be sufficient for current and future IgE-blocking MABs. Administration before the season when more pollen is expected may be worthy of consideration. Doctors may target cough/sputum and mucus production for so-called cough-variant asthma. The remodeling process may produce goblet cell hyperplasia. Known triggers such as NOTCH, SPDEF, and others may represent new therapeutic avenues. Grainge et al. (2011) challenged accepted paradigms by showing that an allergen and nonspecific noninflammatory methacholine could induce goblet cell hyperplasia; it could be prevented by inhaled bronchodilators irrespective of the level of airway inflammation. The remodeling process of chronic airway obstruction in asthma is different from COPD and less understood. Patients' autopsies have shown that airway remodeling results from mucus plugging the small airways and smooth muscle enlargement. Thermoplasty may benefit this condition.

Aspirin and other nonsteroidal anti-inflammatory drugs may trigger asthma by interfering with eicosanoid metabolism. Świerczyńska-Krępa et al. (2014) found that leukotriene receptor antagonists were good candidates for benefiting aspirin tolerance.

Obesity

Few people understand what happens in the body when one has excess weight. Fat cells or adipocytes send out many hormones that affect various bodily functions. When a person is obese and also has asthma, it is most challenging. Studies involving obesity have revealed that asthma and obesity are somewhat related in pathogenesis, but there is still no pharmaceutical strategy for treatment. Yuksel et al. (2012) found that adipokines or hormones involved in fat cells are related to asthma. Steroids, the gold standard treatment for asthma, have been linked to weight gain and may cause a cycle of therapy and excess weight. Marin et al. (2013) showed that small airway abnormities play an essential role in obese people with asthma but did not identify the problem's exact nature. The studies of the impact of bariatric surgery on asthma are not conclusive.

Epigenetics

This topic is the study of heritable changes not caused by changes in the genetic code itself. These mechanisms explain genomic adaption for specific environmental influences and also to the development of the disease. Several known molecular mechanisms are involved in epigenetics, such as DNA methylations, post-transcriptional histone modification, and modification of noncoding RNAs. These mechanisms alter gene expression, which leads to disease expression in different individuals. However, as a study by Kabesch et al. (2010) showed, little is known about the epigenetic mechanism in allergy and asthma; studies are underway. Bell and Saffery (2012) investigated identical twins (monozygotic twins) who have the same genome and tend to have the same environmental influences. The researchers were puzzled when only one twin developed asthma or allergy while the other remained unaffected. They explained that each twin may still have experienced a different microflora environment, environmental tobacco smoke, dietary factors, or traffic exhaust that induced epigenetic expression.

Environmental Control

Politics may have a role in environmental policies to improve respiratory health. Such issues as air pollution, schools being aware of environmental conditions, reducing indoor/outdoor air pollution, and adapting occupational exposure are in people's hands to improve air quality.

IMPROVING DRUG DELIVERY: NANOTECHNOLOGY

Although scientists have made progress in investigating asthma treatments, no single treatment exists due to its complex pathogenesis. However, new hope may be forthcoming with advances in nanotechnology. Nanotechnology is a multidisciplinary field of research, which works with and controls atoms and molecules of very minute size. The particles range from 0.1 to 11 nanometers (nm). Nanoparticles are among the most widely studied drug delivery systems, as described in over 25,000 articles in the past few years. Studies have shown the safety and efficacy of nanocarriers.

The potential of nanotechnology in asthma treatment falls into two categories: traditional molecular drugs improved by nanotechnology and brand-new nanodrugs. These strategies include nanoparticles that carry existing drugs, deliver them to a specific target, reduce side effects, and improve drugs' solubility. Traditional antiasthma drugs are given intravenously, orally, or by inhalation. Improving the drugs with nanoparticles enables inhalation to reach the respiratory target with fewer doses and fewer side effects. New nanodrugs are highly effective with low toxicity. Only a few studies have explored the new nanotherapy for asthma and the abnormal expressions of multiple genes. Nanosized carriers, as the gene transfer vectors, wrap DNA and RNA in nanoparticles. These particles are cutting-edge, with only preclinical studies demonstrating safety and effectiveness. There will be many challenges before practitioners can apply nanotherapy in clinical practice.

CONTROLLING SEVERE ASTHMA; CURING MILD ASTHMA

Excessive chronic airway inflammation characterizes severe asthma. With the inflammation, the host protects itself and returns to homeostasis or resolution. Many substances rush in to resolve inflammation. Novel compounds such as lipozins, protectins, resolvins, and maresins are specialized proresolving mediators (SPMs). Asthma is a heterogeneous disease with many subtypes. Some of the most severe types are not understood. Efforts to control severe asthma and to cure mild asthma are subjects of research.

Allergic Bronchopulmonary Aspergillosis (ABPA)

ABPA is characterized by an exaggerated response of the immune system to the fungus Aspergillus. It sometimes occurs in people with asthma and cystic fibrosis. The condition may be either mild or severe. Treating this condition with antimycotic therapy involves evaluating if the individual risk of treatment outweighs the benefits. Poitiers University Hospital (2015) had success with nebulized formulations of liposomal amphotericin B in treating ABPA. IgE neutralization has also been suggested. Intervention and a better understanding of how mucus plugs the airways, leading to irreversible bronchiectasis, are unmet needs in treating ABPA.

Viruses also require deeper understanding. Rhinoviruses are the most common cause of asthma attacks. According to Caliskan et al. (2013), many researchers have hypothesized that increased asthma is related to the impaired interferon (INF) response to infection. Supplementing this defect with INF helped patients with severe asthma. Researchers suggest that INF could be used as a treatment "as needed."

IMPROVING EXISTING THERAPEUTICS

Scientists are improving the efficacy and efficiency of current options by improving drug delivery, better devices, and new pharmacological families. But the future of treatment lies in the improvement of patient characterization. We will explore the idea of personalized medicine and note the importance of determining clinical characteristics or phenotypes with biomarkers or endotypes. Patients' knowledge and insights may bridge the gap between research and expectations. Addressing the most severe forms of asthma will undoubtedly be a priority. And basic science will provide the mechanisms to achieve the challenges of controlling severe asthma and curing mild asthma.

New Inhaled Corticosteroids (ICS)

Indeed, for the last few decades, ICS has been the gold standard of treatment and has resulted in reduced death, fewer hospital admissions, and improvements worldwide. However, several researchers, including Dahl (2006), described the many side effects: adrenal insufficiency, diabetes, skin bruising, oral mycosis, reduced bone density, and reduced growth in children; fear of these side effects has led to inadequate levels of adherence or mistrust of ICS. Developing new and safer ICS may address these issues. For example, Gaurvreau et al. (2015) found that a nonsteroidal glucocorticoid receptor agonist inhibits allergen-induced late asthmatic responses. Improving drug half-life may be another strategy.

New Long-Acting Beta-Agonists and Long-Acting Muscarinic Agonists (LABAs)

New LABAs have been developed for COPD and might be effective against asthma. Scientists are investigating the potential here, but as of 2020, the effect is unknown.

Inhaled Therapies

Lavorini et al. (2019) reviewed many devices for inhaled therapy. They found a lack of evidence-based guidance for health-care providers and help in choosing the correct inhaler. They discussed the relative merits of selecting the right inhalers and the values of dry powder inhalers, pressurized meter dose inhalers, breath-actuated pressurized metered-dose inhalers, spacers, and soft-mist inhalers. They also investigated the impact of patient perceptions and patient education and emphasized the importance of developing technology in inhaler design and the need for standardized study assessment.

The FDA in 2020 approved the Tevo's AirDuo Digihaler® as digital maintenance for asthma. The device contains a built-in electronic module that records and stores information about inhaler events. AirDuo Digihaler® is a combination of fluticasone propionate, a steroid, and salmeterol, a long-acting LABA. The treatment is designed for patients age 12 and older. This device will give health-care providers the ability to measure patient inspiration flow and track maintenance medication and the inhaler frequency.

2020 FOCUSED UPDATE TO THE ASTHMA MANAGEMENT GUIDELINES

To establish best practices for clinicians and researchers, diverse experts who work in the field have formed a group called the National Asthma Education and Prevention Program Coordinated Committee Expert Panel Working Group. The group had established recommendations in 2007 and in 2020 updated the six topics: Fractional Nitric Oxide tests, indoor allergen mitigation in asthma management, the role of subcutaneous immunotherapy (SCIT) and sublingual immunotherapy (SLIT), bronchial thermoplasty, step therapy, and long-acting muscarinic antagonists as add-ons to inhaled corticosteroids.

The panel recommended SCIT as an adjunct to standard pharmacotherapy.

Fractional Exhaled Nitric Oxide (FeNO)

FeNO is an endogenous gaseous molecule that measures the human breath test for airway inflammation. The panel recommended the use of this test as an adjunct test if a diagnosis is uncertain. It is useful to follow disease activity and medication management with regular testing. Practitioners should not use it as a stand-alone test to assess control, predict future problems, or determine severity.

Further recommendations include considering factors such as ICS, smoking status, age, and allergic sensitization. The data points need to be refined and validated in different ethnic groups and those with comorbidities. This practice should not be a routine office test in primary care settings without strong specialty support.

Indoor Allergen Mitigation in Asthma Management

These suggestions target those with symptoms and sensitization. An integrated strategy for avoidance is recommended, including pest management as a single dose or part of a multicomponent program. Impermeable pillow/mattress covers are essential as part of the strategy. However, the panel did not recommend the mitigation strategy for those not sensitized to a specific allergen. The problem here is that there has been no standardization of outcomes. Although the cost may be small, following these strategies may distract other therapy aspects.

Role of Subcutaneous Immunotherapy (SCIT) and Sublingual Immunotherapy (SLIT)

Doctors can use SCIT in adults and children over the age of five with mild to moderate asthma. Asthma should be under control at the initiation, buildup, and during maintenance of the immunotherapy. The panel recommends against SLIT. For all immunotherapy strategies, the panel recommends the importance of shared decision-making. The benefits of

SCIT appear to be small improvements in symptoms and quality of life or reduction in long-term medications. Although it may improve certain comorbid conditions, there is still the risk of systemic reactions. To optimize control, avoid the treatment with severe asthma and administered only in a clinical setting. In administering SLIT or sublingual therapy, only a limited of allergens have FDA approval for allergic rhinoconjunctivitis. Studies show trivial benefits on critical outcomes in asthma. SLIT may reduce the need for the use of quick-relief and other controlled medication.

Bronchial Thermoplasty

The panel recommended against the use of bronchial thermoplasty, which uses heat to treat smooth airways. They were critical of studies that did not include individuals who received low acting muscarinic agonist (LAMA), environmental interventions, and newer biologic agents. Medicines should be optimized before even considering bronchial thermoplasty and then carefully discuss the risks and benefits with each patient. One group of adults with persistent asthma who place a low value on unknown side effects may consider bronchial thermoplasty. However, it should be considered only in the context of registries or ongoing clinical trials.

Step Therapy

The panel still indicated the Expert Panel Report 3 (EPR-3) as the preferred choice. When alternative options have been developed, they have been shown to be less effective than the select options or have more limited evidence. However, an option may still be useful for some patients.

Adjustable Inhaled Corticosteroid Dosing in Recurrent Wheezing and Asthma

At the onset of a respiratory infection, patients should have a short course of daily ICS with SABA needed for quick relief. Children ages zero through four with recurrent wheezing triggered by respiratory tract infections and not wheezing between infections may use adjustable dosing. Doctors may use it in children ages zero through four who have had three or more wheezing episodes triggered by respiratory infections in their lifetime or two in the past year. Not recommended is a short-term increase in the ICS dose for increased symptoms or decreased peak flow. The procedure is not recommended for children ages four years old and older who are likely to adhere to daily ICS treatment. A short-term increase in ICS is defined as doubling, quadrupling, or quintupling the regular daily dose.

Long-Acting Muscarinic Antagonists as Add-On to Inhaled Corticosteroids

Either daily low-dose ICS and SABA for quick relief should be given as needed. The experts recommend SMART Maintenance and Reliever therapy.

The panel considered and discussed the following topics: prevention of asthma, biomarkers other than FeNO, asthma severity classification, biologics, asthma treatment plans, the role of community health workers, asthma heterogeneity including endotypes and phenotypes, adherence, LABA safety, and step down from maintenance therapy.

PERSONALIZED MEDICINE AND THE FUTURE

Most health-care professionals proclaim that personalized medicine will be the wave of the future. Researchers worldwide are working to solve how genes and lifestyle connect to affect our lives and health and how medicine can meet individuals' needs. It all relates to the individual's genetic makeup. Now, groups can scan and compare entire genomes very quickly. The Human Genome Project and thousands of other studies help scientists develop gene-targeted treatments, not only for asthma but also for many other diseases, such as type 2 diabetes, heart disorders, and prostate cancers.

More Disease-Related Gene Variants

Researchers are identifying more disease-related variants every few months. Thanks to such agencies as the National Institutes of Health and other groups, research has given us genetic engineering and launched a $40 billion biotech industry. DNA is now a household name. Many people have their genomes analyzed through popular sites like 23andMe or ancestry.com.

One can imagine how sequencing the genome might eventually be used in the clinic. For example, a recent NIH study showed how the scientists evaluated a 40-year-old man's entire genome to determine his risk for dozens of diseases and response to standard drugs. Remarkable pharmacogenomics advances show that individuals react differently to medicine and indicate we are moving away from "one-size-fits-all" medications. Some drugs may be dangerous or even ineffective for certain people. Also, the information will help doctors calculate precise dosages that match the person's DNA.

The area of biomedicine will prompt the FDA to change the labeling requirements for essential medicines. Pharmacogenomics information is already contained in about 10% of labels for all drugs. So we can imagine the future using a patient's genetic profile—not just weight or age—to determine the best medicine and optimal dose.

Another area relating to personalized medicine is the promise of stem cells for biomedical science. Stem cells may lead to cell-based therapies for many conditions that affect Americans.

Personalized Medicine and Pharmacogenetics

Asthma is a chronic inflammatory disease associated with airway hyper-responsiveness, chronic inflammatory response, and excessive structural remodeling. The goal of personalized medicine is to predict which patients will respond to any treatment. Based on genetic polymorphisms, doctors will be able to individualize drug treatment for those who are most likely to react and avoid those treatments that might be harmful. Candidate genes are those that encode receptor proteins and enzymes involved in drug transportation, processing, degradation, and excretion. For example, Slager et al. (2010) found that in an experimental drug blocking the IL-4/IL-13 pathway, individual amino acid variations in the IL-4 receptor appeared to predict which patients would have the best treatment response of increased lung function.

Personalizing medicine is much more complicated than at first glance. The biological pathways that form the basis of the different kinds of asthma called endotypes are based on the Th2/non-Th-2 paradigm, but identifying the Th2 endotype is not simple. The potential now lies within the analysis of sputum samples and blood eosinophil count. After the analysis, finding the drug to match the endotype is the challenge.

Researchers are investigating the endotypes Th2 vs. non-Th2. Most drugs are currently being developed as target Th2 cytokines. Th2 cytokines and their receptors and Th2 cells have all been targeted. These targets include interleukin (IL)-4, IL-5, IL-9, IL-13, IL-23, IL-25, IL-33, IgE, and thymic stromal lymphopoietin (TSLP); others will be targeted in the future. The non-Th2 types are not well understood, and the investigation is limited.

Some strategies are potentially used to target the clinical characteristics of asthma. In order to personalize treatment, atopy is probably the first phenotypic trait for the target. Atopy refers to the genetic tendency to develop allergic diseases such as rhinitis, asthma, and eczema. Avoidance and immunotherapy are two cornerstones of the management, and adding a rescue drug such as omalizumab may still be insufficient. New outlooks on the anti-IgE blockade may improve IgE binding. Gauvreau et al. (2014) found that the optimal frequency of administration of quilizumab may be effective for current and future IgE-blocking MABs. Administration before the worsening season, the season when more pollen is in the air, may be of worthwhile consideration. Cough/sputum and mucus production may be targeted for so-called cough-variant asthma. The remodeling process may produce goblet cell hyperplasia. Known triggers such as NOTCH, SPDEF, and others may represent new therapeutic avenues. Grainge et al. (2011) challenged accepted paradigms by showing that goblet cell hyperplasia could be induced but can emerge with an allergen and nonspecific noninflammatory methacholine; it could be prevented inhaled bronchodilators irrespective of the level of airway inflammation. The remodeling process of chronic airway obstruction in asthma is different from COPD and less understood. Patients' autopsies have shown that airway remodeling results from mucus plugging or the small airways and smooth muscle enlargement. Thermoplasty may benefit this condition.

Aspirin and other nonsteroidal anti-inflammatory drugs may trigger asthma by interfering with eicosanoid metabolism. Świerczyńska-Krępa et al. (2014) found that leukotriene receptor antagonists were good candidates for benefiting aspirin tolerance.

STEM CELLS AND ASTHMA

Stem cells are often talked about but poorly misunderstood. Stem cells are specific cells that have the potential to replicate themselves and are of basically two kinds: embryonic stem cells and adult stem cells. The classification is based not on the location but on the stage of development. Mesenchymal stem cells (MSCs) are those taken from body tissues, especially in the abdominal area.

Investigation of stem cells generally targets the pulmonary tissue. Current therapeutic strategies for asthma are based on the control in type 2 helper lymphocytes in the pulmonary tissue; however, most of these therapies are expensive, with diverse side effects. To date, different reports have highlighted the benefits of transplantation of stem cell sources. When these procedures are better understood, stem cells can then translate into the clinical setting. Mirershadi et al. (2020) reviewed the current knowledge and future perspective related to the therapeutic applications regarding animal models of asthma. It seems that adult bone marrow stem cells, which are MSCs, have regenerative potential. MSCs have been prominent in several experimental studies. They are correlated with the immune system at the inflammation site and are eligible to recalculate the Th2 to Th1 ratio, synthesis of interleukins such as 4, 5 and 13, IGE, and mucus.

The study concluded that MSC delivery could diminish inflammation of the lungs and airway conduits in asthmatic animal models. However, as of December 2020, understanding the exact mechanism of MSC-therapy is mandatory before clinicians can use stem cells. The exact bioactivity of MSCs is still unclear and continues to be investigated.

CONCLUSION

The future of a disease like asthma is undoubtedly very complex. We can see from the long list of topics the panel had to consider that decisions about the nature of care and future directions are challenging. We presented several research areas, including disease modifiers, new immunotherapies, behavioral modifications (mainly involving the microbiome), genetics and personalized medicine, environmental control, improving existing therapies, and improving drug delivery through nanotechnology. We have looked at the efforts to control severe asthma and cure mild asthma. Indeed, not all of these future efforts will ever reach the clinic. Many pharmaceutical agents will come and go as others replace them. However, we do conclude that the general premise will be personalized medicine. This approach will bring in researchers, patients, clinicians, and the industry. The answers are not there yet, and still, there are lots of questions. But the future of research is bright and hopeful. The challenge here is to bring together biology and practicality.

Case Studies

BAKERY BLUES

Jeannette decided to take a year off between high school and college. She felt that having the extra time would help her decide what she wanted to do and give her the money she needed for college. In the local newspaper, she read that the most prestigious bakery in town was hiring and wanted dependable people. This placement would not be her first job. She had worked at the local supermarket and was reliable and hardworking.

The interview went flawlessly. In this bakery job, she would be the mixer and work for four hours a day. Another colleague would bring her the flour and other ingredients. She would pour them into the large blender and set the timer. It was thrilling to pour the flour into the large vessel and watch the flume of flour rise. She would turn her head for a quick cough and then continue to pour in the sugar and other ingredients that would become cookies, cakes, and other goodies.

The first couple of days were great. Jeannette felt very good about her new job and even was able to bring home some samples. However, on the third day, she noted that her nose was itching. Later, that day she noted shortness of breath, coughing, wheezing, and chest tightening. The symptoms continued for days.

Interestingly, when she left work and had been out of the building for a while, she appeared to be better, but still, at times, the cough and wheezing continued.

She decided that it was getting into cold weather and that this must be a seasonal cold. However, the cold did not go away. She finally decided to go to Dr. Smith, her family doctor. Not knowing that she was working in the bakery, he gave her medication and told her to rest. Being at home for a few days helped, and she felt much better. So she went back to work after a week.

The coughing and wheezing began again. This time, she told Dr. Smith that she was working at the best bakery in town. He now was quite sure he knew what this was but sent her to Dr. Bunker, the allergy specialist, for a consultation.

Dr. Bunker performed a skin prick test and an allergen serology study. The skin test involved cleaning Jeannette's forearm and marking off the area into 40 tiny spaces. He pricked the skin with a small sample taken from 40 different vials. This test checked for immediate reactions to allergens. He performed a second test called an allergen serology study. In this test, the person gives a blood sample. The doctor can measure the levels of antibodies called immunoglobulin E (IgE) against specific allergens such as foods, inhalants, dust mites, or other substances. The enzyme-linked immunoassay (ELISA) has generally replaced an older blood test called the radioallergosorbent test (RAST).

Through the tests, the doctors found that Jeanette had three allergies: wheat flour, various additives such as amylase and cellulose, and dust mites. They referred to it as baker's asthma. She was surprised that the plume of flour had caused her to cough, and she did not realize that certain additives to help the product knead more easily were a problem. And what was the origin of these dust mites? She found out when she went into the storage room and saw that a thick layer of dust covered the stacks of sacks.

The doctors prescribed an inhaler for her immediate issues but told her that she must wear a mask around these products if she wanted to work in the bakery. They also talked to the bakery owners about provisions for other workers and about cleaning the dust in storage rooms often.

Jeannette worked for one year at the bakery with a few other incidents. She then decided to attend community college. She is still aware that she must be very cautious whenever she is around flour, even in her kitchen. That impressive flume may cause a latent reaction.

Analysis

Bernardino Ramazzini (1633–1714), the father of occupational medicine, always asked his patients, "What is your occupation?" Some early writers in 1713 recorded reports of a severe breathing condition among those milling and baking. These people experienced shortness of breath, hoarseness, cough, and wheezing. An ancient condition, baker's asthma, one of the first described occupational diseases, continues as a problem to this day. The underlying causes were diagnosed in the 1970s and 1980s when immunological techniques were developed.

It appears that the problem arises not only from flour but also from the amylase enzyme, a dough conditioner added to flour to improve the quality of the product. This enzyme comes from the organism *Aspergillus oryzae*, which, when added to flour, compensates for low natural amylase levels in cereal flour.

To minimize the level of flour dust, additives, and other asthma-causing agents inhaled by bakery workers, medical professionals and restaurant leaders should consider the following:

- provide face masks to employees;
- incorporate housekeeping tasks like wet scrubbing and vacuuming surfaces;
- control the amount of flour dust by enclosing dusty machinery or installing local exhaust ventilation; and
- employ dough-mixing approaches that reduce the amount of dust generated.

The worst thing that can happen is to dump out a flour bag and generate a large plume of dust.

ALL IN THE HOUSE

Four-year-old Zach, an energetic preschool student, had one great interest: dinosaurs. He could tell you everything about Tyrannosaurus rex and Triceratops. He loved to go to school but kept getting colds and having to miss school. Even when his cold symptoms disappeared, he coughed quite a bit at night. Occasionally, his parents heard him wheezing at night. They also noticed that he had some trouble breathing or breathed so rapidly that the skin around the ribs or neck would pull in tightly. But on one occasion, it was different. He almost stopped breathing. His frightened parents called 911, and the ambulance rushed him to the emergency room. The emergency doctors told them that it was probably an asthma attack, and after the emergency treatment, they should take the boy to his pediatrician.

Dr. Morse, his pediatrician, comforted his mom, who was known as a real helicopter mom, responding to the slightest discomfort her son may show. Dr. Morse explained to the frightened parents how the passageways that allowed air to enter and leave the lungs were small and narrow. If the child had a head cold or chest cold, it could inflame the airways and make them even smaller. He also told them how hard it was for parents and even doctors to recognize asthma symptoms. He explained that making a diagnosis is difficult because the first type of test—the airflow test—is almost impossible to do with young children. He asked for permission to do a skin test to find the source of his irritants.

Dr. Morse also probed into what may be happening at home. The parents described how their house was insulated and airtight and cozy and warm during the winter. Zach only went out to get into the car to go to school. Although both parents admitted that they smoked, they made it clear that they refrained from smoking around the boy or in his room. That was a red flag. Dr. Morse found one of the possible triggers for Zack's attacks: thirdhand smoke. Although they were careful not to smoke in the house, the odor lingered on their clothing and hair and could irritate young lungs.

The skin test revealed four other irritants that could make the symptoms worse: pollen, mold, pet dander, and dust mites. Mom was shocked at the suggestion of dust and tiny mites in her house until Dr. Morse pointed out that these mites can stay in the carpet, upholstered furniture, and their favorite artificial silk plants. The family also had a pet cat named Toby. They felt that their airtight house does not let in things like pollen from the outside. They found that mold was everywhere. Even the air ducts that heated the house may be blowing mold around.

The doctor prescribed asthma medication, and the family worked out an asthma plan for prevention. They would detail the house to control dust by vacuuming walls and furniture often. Vacuuming would also aid in the control of dust mites. Grandmother would take Toby, the cat. The couple agreed to go to smoking cessation classes. They also developed a plan for how to look for symptoms and how to use and take medication. The program included how to instruct the teachers at school and when to seek emergency help.

Zack is now five. The parents have been very conscientious in following the written plan. They have it posted on their refrigerator to remind them how frightened they were and that now they are in command. He has not had an attack or a cold in several months.

Analysis

Childhood asthma is the most common severe chronic disease in infants and children. It is difficult to diagnose as it may appear as a cold, a whistling sound, coughing, or rapid breathing. To correctly manage the condition, the physician must make a proper diagnosis, and the parents must make changes in the home environment.

As the doctor pointed out, proper diagnosis presents unique challenges in preschool children. They will probably be unable to complete the airflow test, which requires the child to blow very hard into a tube. And young children may not be able to describe how they feel. The onus is on the parents, family members, and caregivers to know the signs and symptoms of asthma.

Changing the indoor environment can be quite a challenge, especially with regard to dust and dust mites. According to the ALA, roughly four out of five homes in the United States have detectable levels of dust mite allergens in at least one bed. Mold is also a household problem. Molds may lead to allergic sensitization and asthma. Researchers say that at least 60 species of molds are thought to be allergenic. According to a study by Etzel (2003), children are most sensitive to mold allergens.

Exposure to environmental tobacco smoke is a severe risk factor for asthma. The EPA has found over 4,000 different tobacco smoke chemicals, with more than 50 being probable causes of cancer. Especially vulnerable are growing children and unborn babies. Thirdhand smoke is also a severe hazard for people with asthma. When one smokes a cigarette, chemicals stick to the surface and dust for months after the smoke is gone. People who are very young and very old are especially at risk for these types of particles, which may be worse for those with asthma than nicotine.

COUNTRY ROADS, 1945

It was 1945, and the state had finally agreed to pave some of rural Mississippi's dusty roads. The citizens of the town would soon be connected to the modern world. Many tractors, steam shovels, and dump trucks hauled dirt and limestone to make the road. Although the idea of the new road was exciting, no one minded the white dust that covered the whole town. Ten-year-old Charles and his friends were fascinated by the road-building process and spent hours watching and running after the machines. They did not mind the dust. Charles and his friends even set up a lemonade stand near the construction site to serve the workers.

It seemed to happen mostly at night. Almost every night, Charles woke up telling his parents that he felt like he was breathing through a straw. He would wheeze and cough. He would even lie on the floor, gasping for air. When these attacks occurred, his parents panicked. In this small, rural town in Mississippi, Dr. Tisdale, the only physician for miles around, still did house calls. He took out his strip of newspaper and carefully rolled up doses of chamomile for Charles to take. This treatment did not help.

Fortunately, his parents had the funds to take him to an allergy specialist in Memphis, 300 miles away. After hearing about the symptoms and listening to his chest, Dr. Brown did a series of tiny pinpricks on Charles's back. Because his back was so broad, he could do them all at one time. The tests revealed he had allergies, and one especially to dust. For two years, the family took Charles to a doctor in the county seat who gave him allergy shots. At that time, knowledge about allergies and asthma was in its infancy.

The allergy specialist set up very rigid rules for the family to follow. The home environment must be kept as free from dust as possible, and Charles had to give up watching the construction of the road and his lemonade stand. He slept on a rubber sheet and pillow, and his parents had to clean the walls and floors of the room each day. After two years, the road was completed, and Charles appeared to have conquered asthma.

Charles overcame asthma, but throughout his adult life, he had some associated incidents with his immune system. When living on a farm in rural Florida, he helped his children with a 4-H project by hauling large sacks of corn for their cattle to consume. That night he started gasping for air, and large white welts called hives covered the arms and stomach where the corn dander had touched. One day for dinner, his wife fixed a Chinese dish with unknown spices; his throat immediately began to close up, and the white welts developed on his neck and back. Benadryl kept him from going into anaphylactic shock.

When he developed an annoying skin condition on the palms of his hands, he went to the dermatologist, who asked him if he had asthma at any time during his life. Of course, the answer was yes, when he was 10. The dermatologist mentioned that his reactions were functions of the immune system and called the condition atopic dermatitis. At least the breathing issues have not appeared again. He does not have to carry bags of corn anymore and does not eat Chinese food.

Analysis

Knowledge and treatment of asthma and allergies have come a long way since the days when Charles had his shots. Constructing roads in the 1940s was a great help to people; however, construction dust can damage the health of individuals who live near the roads. As building roads and even construction projects take a long time, regular breathing of harmful dust can be life-threatening.

Today, in many areas of the country, new infrastructure is being constructed. Anyone who works with construction dust or lives in areas near the original buildings or new roads should know the risks to their health. Asthma may come on quickly. In addition to asthma, other dust-related diseases are lung cancer, silicosis, and COPD.

Fortunately, laws today help to control exposure to dangerous situations. The Control of Substances Hazardous to Health Regulation 2002, a.k.a. COSHH, covers activities that may expose workers to construction dust. However, these laws do not apply to people living near construction or doing home projects such as tearing down old structures or driveways. It is up to individuals to keep away from the hazards of breathing plumes of dust from any source.

TROUBLE IN THE ELEMENTARY SCHOOL

Ten-year-old Juan recently moved to Florida from New York. His relatives came from the island of Puerto Rico, but Juan was born on the mainland in the United States. He was in the fourth grade and hated school. He felt the school in New York was terrible, but the one in Florida was even worse. At least in New York, many children could speak Spanish. He was failing all of his subjects.

Juan had significant issues with the other students. They did not like him and called him names like "Fatso" and "Fatty." However, weight was not his primary problem. In class, he had "spells" when he could not breathe; he would grab his chest and gasp for breath. The teacher thought he was seeking attention and sent him to the school clinic. The person in charge of the clinic agreed and sent him back to class. These visits happened over and over. During a "spell," he would cough, wheeze, and grab his chest. It was alarming to his classmates, who rolled their eyes at him. The teacher told him his coughing was disrupting her teaching. However, he did have a favorite time of the day: lunch. He would eat his lunch and finish the plates of all the other students who would give them to him. One teacher reported that she saw him take food from the garbage cans.

During one trip to the clinic, the "nurse" (a paraprofessional who handles sick kids) called his mother at work at the restaurant. His mother told the school she would not come to get him and that he did this all the time at home just to get attention. His parents did not show up for school conferences, and so he only went to school when they sent him and played sick on other days.

A guidance counselor became concerned about the parents' lack of interest in the boy and contacted the Department of Children and Family for possible child neglect. The investigation proved to be enlightening. Both the mother and her live-in boyfriend worked two jobs, and Juan, an only child, was left by himself a lot. The adults did provide lots of food for him, especially peanut butter and crackers and cookies. His mother loved the boy but thought that his weight problem came from his *abuela* (grandmother), who was also very heavy. She also said that *abuela* had spells when she could not breathe, but she thought that *abuela* just needed attention. *Abuela* died two years ago of a lung infection.

Ms. Wise, the caseworker from DCF, now had some clues to this multifaceted problem and how they can solve these issues. It would not be easy. She suspected that asthma caused the breathing "spells." Asthma is very prominent among inhabitants of Puerto Rico and those in the U.S. population who moved here. She also realized that there was a possible connection between his obesity and asthma.

She convinced the parents to take the boy to a children's medical service, and he met Dr. Guadier, also from Puerto Rico, who took a particular interest in Juan. First, he worked with the caregivers and educated them about the condition and its relationship to Juan's physical and educational problems. They were interested and willing to help. An allergy specialist tested Juan and found several things in the home that might cause asthma; he made suggestions on correcting these problems. Juan then began work with a weight-loss specialist, who helped the parents create a nutrition and exercise program for him.

Next, the school had to be involved. Medical professionals would educate teachers and administrators about asthma and its symptoms. The team also agreed to refer Juan for special education services.

Today, Juan has lost 50 pounds and is getting along better with his school peers. He has an inhaler, which stays in the clinic for when he needs it. His school performance is not stellar, but he is much happier. He is still left alone often but now does his exercises at home and stays away from the cookies and peanut butter.

Analysis

This case history is multifaceted, involving Juan and his self-image, the caregivers and home, and the school. Juan's situation is unfortunate. According to studies by the National Institutes of Health, the prevalence of asthma in the United States is higher among Puerto Ricans (16.1%) than in non-Hispanic Blacks (11.2%) and non-Hispanic whites (7.7%). The fact that *abuela* (grandmother) had symptoms was not surprising. If the mother had looked into other relatives, she probably would have found the same thing.

Juan's weight is an initial problem. Finding someone who will help the caregivers understand and help him find the motivation for diet change and exercise will also address his serious health problems. According to the ALA, the excess weight around the chest and abdomen constricts the lungs and makes it harder to breathe. Juan and his parents worked with a weight-loss specialist who set up a plan for lifestyle changes. The allergist addressed his medical problems by giving him proper medication and specific instructions on using the inhaler.

Next, the issues at school might be more challenging to address. Members of the school staff were not aware that a problem existed; the teacher expressed that the "spells" were to get attention. The caseworker from DCF met with the school and teachers. She explained his medical condition and then worked out a plan to get Juan tested for special education with an individual education plan (IEP). Juan found that his weight loss also helped him with his peers. He was no longer called "Fatso."

RUNNING TRACK

Don is an energetic high school student who must choose a sport as part of the International Baccalaureate (IB) program. He likes swimming and baseball but considering the amount of time that must be devoted to these sports, they are not feasible. So, when someone mentioned running track, he thought it might be just for him.

The IB program is very demanding, and Don does have to spend many hours studying, writing, and researching. When he interviewed the coach, he found you do not have to be "fast," and running track may be a perfect place for newbies who have to budget their time between studies and other activities. So, just as he worked so diligently in the IB program, Don jumped into track with enthusiasm, determined to do his best. He learned the lingo of the track and found that the inside lane is for the fastest runners. If you are cooling down or running slowly, choose an outer lane.

His coach started the runners out slowly and then began to increase the number of laps around the track. With the first increase, Don noted shortness of breath. Only reasonable, he thought, because this was something he had not done. But with increased running, he noted two new symptoms: wheezing and coughing. A friend told him that running was causing the shortness of breath, and he would just get over it if he increased his vitamin C intake. However, he did not get over it; it worsened.

In addition to being a very conscientious student, Don was careful about his diet, and he tried to get some exercise by going to the gym. He had studied the respiratory system in biology and knew the basic structure of the respiratory system, with the airway passages from mouth to the trachea, to the bronchi, and then ending in the alveoli in the lungs. From his studies of biology, Don could explain the oxygen–carbon dioxide exchange. However, he knew very little about the lungs' conditions, such as asthma, pneumonia, or COPD.

When Don continued to complain about his shortness of breath and coughing during running, his parents made an appointment with Dr. Balducci, a specialist in sports medicine and related conditions. The doctor was very interested in Don's case. After an intensive case history and learning of the symptoms, the doctor asked permission to perform several tests.

Like most high school athletes, Don had no idea that his cough and hyperventilation were due to the exercised-induced asthma, or EIA. The allergist explained how running is the most effective way to provoke asthma and bronchoconstriction because it is a constant activity. If one plays football or baseball, there is lots of downtime during the innings. This respite does not happen in running track. He also explained that when the athletes get to his office, they appear normal because they have been running or doing the sport, and the signs disappear. To make the diagnosis, he had Don run on a treadmill for 10 minutes. He also administered a spirometry test to assess how well the lungs functioned when Don was not exercising. This test measures how much air you inhale, how much you exhale, and how quickly you exhale. He then gave Don an inhaled medication called a bronchodilator to see if this improved the airflow.

Dr. Balducci told him that runners have many treatment options. The medications are safe, and you can continue to do what you want to do. The doctor laughed and said, "We do not tell you not to run, but we tell you how to run." He recommended that Don use an inhaler 15 to 30 minutes before the race. He also told him never to share his inhaler or use the inhaler of another. The medications were designed specifically for him. He advised him to return if he found this procedure was not working.

Don has been running track for three years now and follows the advice of his doctors carefully. He will probably never be the greatest long-distance runner. Still, his EIA experience has taught him about this and other sports activities that he can participate in throughout his life.

Analysis

There is a lot of mythology about exercise and asthma, and Don's friends were not short on advice. He did have exercise-induced bronchospasms (EIB), the new name for exercise-induced asthma.

Running is probably the most effective way to provoke asthma, exacerbated by inhaling cold, dry air or allergens. With EIB, there is some underlying allergy that is often mild and undetected in the average person. The allergy may cause the bronchial tubes to inflame slightly, but distance running irritates the slight inflammation and causes a spasm. If a person with an allergy runs, he or she will have an issue.

The first meeting with the doctor introduced Don to EIB. He would learn more about it in future visits. Before an event, he would try the inhaler for 15 to 30 minutes, and the effects would last three to four hours. Later, if this treatment was not sufficient, he might receive long-term treatments, such as inhaled corticosteroids, to control the symptoms.

Don's doctor gave him good advice on mitigating the spasms and what to do as he participated in the sport. He may not win a championship, but he does like participating in track meets against other high schools.

Glossary

Airway obstruction
Something that blocks the airways that carry oxygen to the lungs. These substances vary and can arise from the body, like mucus, or from an object that may cause choking.

Allergen
A foreign substance (such as food or pollen) that evokes an immune reaction.

Allergic rhinitis
Inflammation of the nasal passage when coming in contact with specific allergens. Many of these reactions are seasonal.

Allergy
A reaction of the immune system to substances that are harmless to most people. Allergies may vary and may be evoked by food, dust mites, pollen, and other substances.

Alveoli
Small sacs located at the end of the airways in the lungs where oxygen–carbon dioxide exchange takes place

Anaphylaxis
A medical emergency involving an acute allergic reaction. These reactions are serious as a person may go into shock.

Antibiotic
Medication used to treat an infection caused by bacteria. These medications do not protect against viruses, such as those causing the common cold.

Antibody
A protein made in the by plasma cells to neutralize an antigen. When the body forms a specific type known as IgE, an allergic response may occur when the person is exposed again to the allergen.

Anticholinergics
A type of medicine that relaxes the muscle bands, which tighten around the airways. This action opens the airways, letting more air out of the lungs to improve breathing. Anticholinergics also help clear mucus from the lungs.

Antigen
A substance, also called an allergen, which can trigger an immune response. Many allergens are foreign proteins.

Anti-inflammatory
A medication that reduces the symptoms of inflammation, such as airway swelling and mucus production.

Asthma
An inflammatory lung disease of the airways or branches of the lungs (bronchial tubes) that carry air. Asthma causes the airways to narrow, the lining of the airways to swell, and the cells that line the airways to produce more mucus. Symptoms include cough, shortness of breath, wheezing, chest tightness, and excess mucus production. Episodes can be triggered by allergens, infection, exercise, cold air, or other factors.

Atopic dermatitis
A skin condition also known as eczema and characterized by extreme itching. Refer to allergic contact dermatitis.

Bacteria
Organisms that may cause sinusitis, bronchitis, or pneumonia.

Basophil
A type of white blood cell.

Beta-agonists (B-agonists)
Medications that opens the airways of the lung by relaxing the muscles around the airways that have tightened. These medications may be short-acting (quick relief) or long-acting (control).

Bronchial tubes
Airways in the lung that branch from the trachea or windpipe.

Bronchioles
The smallest branches of the airways in the lungs. They connect to the alveoli or air sacs, where the oxygen–carbon dioxide exchange takes place.

Bronchitis
An inflammation of the bronchi, resulting in coughing. The condition is common in smokers and in areas of high air pollution.

Bronchodilators
A group of drugs that that open the airways and relax the muscle bands that tighten around the airways. Bronchodilators help clear mucus from the lungs.

Bronchospasm
The tightening of the muscle bands that surround the airways, causing the airways to narrow.

Carbon dioxide
A colorless, odorless gas formed in the tissues and delivered to the lungs to be exhaled.

Chronic disease
A disease that can be controlled but not cured. At present, asthma cannot be cured but can be controlled or managed.

Cilia
Tiny hairlike projections that line the airways in the lungs. Cilia help clean out the airways.

Clinical trials
Research programs conducted with patients to evaluate a new medical treatment, drug, or device. There are three phases that new treatments must go through before the U.S. Food and Drug Administration approves it for use.

Corticosteroid drugs
A group of anti-inflammatory medications similar to natural hormones produced in the cortex of the adrenal glands. These drugs are used to treat asthma.

Cytokines
A group of protein molecules that cells release in response to activation or injury.

Dander, animal
Tiny scales from animal skin or hair. Dander is a common allergen that floats in the air, settles on surfaces, and is a major part of household dust.

Dehydration
Excessive loss of water. Dehydration is dangerous when it reaches the cellular level.

Diaphragm
The major muscle of breathing. It is located at the base of the lungs.

Dry powder inhaler (DPI)
A device for inhaling medications that come in powder form.

Dust mites
Microscopic animals found in dust. These mites are a common trigger for allergies.

Eczema
An inflammation of the skin, characterized by itching, crusting, or blisters. Eczema is also called atopic dermatitis.

Eosinophil
A type of white blood cells which may modulate immune responses. High levels are present in some kinds of asthma.

Epinephrine
A naturally occurring hormone also called adrenaline.

Exacerbation
Worsening.

Exercise-induced asthma
Asthma that is made worse when exercising. Certain types of exercise such as running or exercising in cold weather may cause this condition.

Hay fever
Inflammation of the mucous membranes of the nose. It is also known as allergic rhinitis.

High-efficiency particulate air filter (HEPA)
A filter that removes particles in the air by forcing it through screens containing microscopic pores. These filters are used in vacuum cleaners.

Histamine
A naturally occurring chemical released by the immune system after being exposed to an allergen. When you inhale an allergen, mast cells located in the nose and lungs release histamine. Histamine also binds to other receptors located in nasal tissues, causing redness, swelling, itching, and changes in the secretions.

Hives
An allergic skin reaction characterized by small itchy bumps or blisters.

Holding chamber
See spacer.

Hydrofluoroalkane inhaler (HFA)
Small aerosol canister in a plastic container that releases a mist of medication when pressed down from the top. This drug can be breathed into the airways.

Hyperventilation
Excessive rate and depth of breathing.

Immune system
The body's defense system that protects us against infections and foreign substances.

Immunoglobulin
Also known as antibodies. These substances are produced by B-lymphocytes. An example is Immunoglobulin E, or IgE, the primary antibody responsible for allergic reactions.

Indication
Reason to use.

Inflammation
A response in the body that may include swelling and redness. It is characteristic of allergic reactions in the nose, eyes, lungs, and skin.

Inhaler
See hydrofluoroalkane inhaler (HFA).

Irritants
Things that bother the nose, throat, or airways when they are inhaled. These are not allergens.

Leukotrienes
Naturally occurring substances in the body that cause tightening of airway muscles and production of excess mucus and fluid. Leukotriene modifiers work by blocking leukotrienes and decreasing these reactions. These medications may also be helpful in improving airflow and reducing some symptoms of asthma.

Lymphocyte
A group of white blood cells that is important in the immune system. These substances mount a defense against foreign invaders.

Mast cells
Cells that play an important part in the immune response. They are present in most tissues but especially numerous in connective tissue.

Metered-dose inhaler (MDI)
See hydrofluoroalkane inhaler (HFA).

Mold
Microscopic fungi with spores that float in the air like pollen. Mold, a common trigger for allergies, can be found in damp areas, such as the basement or bathroom, as well as in the outdoor environment in grass, leaf piles, hay, mulch, or under mushrooms.

Monitoring
Keeping track of.

Mucus
A substance produced by glands in the airways, nose, and sinuses. Mucus cleans and protects certain parts of the body, such as the lungs.

Nebulizer
A device that changes liquid medicine into fine droplets. A nebulizer may be used instead of a metered-dose inhaler (MDI). It is powered by a compressed air machine and plugs into an electrical outlet.

Non-steroidal
An anti-inflammatory medication that is not a steroid. Also see steroid.

Occupational asthma
Asthma that is contracted by breathing fine dust or fumes that result from the job. An example is "bakers' asthma," common in people who work around flour.

Otitis media
Middle ear infection common in infants and children with allergic rhinitis. This also may be referred to as "earache."

Oxygen
The essential element in the respiration process to sustain life. This colorless, odorless gas makes up about 21% of the air.

Peak expiratory flow rate
A test used to measure how fast air can be exhaled from the lungs.

Peak flow meter
A small handheld device that measures air speed coming out of the lungs when a person exhales. Readings from the meter can help the patient recognize early changes that may be signs of worsening asthma. A peak flow meter can also help patients learn what triggers their symptoms and understand what symptoms indicate that emergency care is needed. Peak flow readings also help the doctor decide when to stop or add medications.

Pneumonia
An infection of the lung that can be caused by bacteria, a virus, or a fungus.

Pollen
A fine, powdery substance released by plants and trees; an allergen. Pollen is the male fertilizing agent of flowering plants, trees, grasses, and weeds.

Productive cough
A "wet" cough that may involve coughing up mucus.

Respiratory system
The group of organs involved in the process of breathing. The system includes mouth, trachea, bronchi, and lungs. See inhalation and exhalation.

Sensitization
The repeated exposure to a foreign substance that makes the person susceptible to an allergic reaction.

Sinuses
Air pockets inside the bones of the head and face that link to the nose.

Spacer
A chamber that is used with a metered-dose inhaler to help the medication get into the airways better. Spacers also make metered-dose inhalers easier to use; spacers are sometimes called "holding chambers."

Spirometry
A basic pulmonary function test that measures how much and how fast air moves out of the lungs.

Sputum
Mucus or phlegm.

Steroid
Medication that reduces swelling and inflammation. Steroids may be in pill form, injected, and inhaled. Also called corticosteroid.

Symptom
What someone will experience as a result of a disease or illness. Symptoms of asthma include wheezing, shortness of breath, and an inability to breath properly.

Theophylline
A long-term control medication that opens the airways, which helps prevent and relieve bronchospasms.

Trachea
The main airway (windpipe) supplying both lungs.

Triggers
Things that cause asthma symptoms to begin or make them worse. Asthma has many triggers for an attack.

Vaccine
A shot that protects the body from a specific disease by stimulating the body's immune system.

Wheezing
A high-pitched, whistling sound of air moving through narrowed airways.

Directory of Resources

BOOKS

Berger, William. (2011). *Asthma for Dummies and a Reference for the Rest of Us.* New York: Wiley.

Chen, Wendy, and Izzy Bean. (2015). *I Have Asthma, What Does That Mean?* Burke, VA: Wendy Chen Books.

Fanta, Christopher, et al. (2007). *The Asthma Educator's Handbook.* New York: McGraw-Hill.

Global Initiative for Asthma. (2019). *Pocket Guide for Asthma Management and Prevention.* Fontana-on-Geneva Lake, WI: Global Initiative for Asthma.

Hannaway, Paul. (2002). *Asthma—An Emerging Epidemic.* Marblehead, MA: Lighthouse Press.

Hogshed, Nancy. (1990). *Asthma and Exercise.* New York: Holt and Company.

Mahmoudi, Massoud. (2008). *Allergy and Asthma: Practical Diagnosis and Management.* New York: McGraw Hill.

Mahmoudi, Massoud. (2017). *Allergy and Asthma Made Ridiculously Simple (Made Ridiculously Simple: Rapid Learning and Retention).* New York: Medmaster, Inc.

Marlo, Coleen (narrator). (2020). *Allergies, Asthma, and the Common Cold.* Ashland, OR: An audio-book published by Scientific American and Blackstone.

Plaut, Thomas. (1998). *One Minute Asthma: What You Need to Know.* Amherst, MA. www.pedipress.com.

Plaut, Thomas F. (1999). *Dr. Thomas Plaut's Asthma Guide for People of All Ages.* Amherst, MA. www.pedipress.com.

Sander, Nancy. (1994). *A Parent's Guide to Asthma: How You Can Help Your Child Control Asthma at Home.* New York: Plume/Penguin.

Wray, Betty. (1997). *Taking Charge of Asthma*. New York: John Wiley and Sons.

ONLINE ARTICLES AND RESOURCES

Agency for Healthcare Research and Quality. "Characteristics of Existing Asthma Self-management." https://effectivehealthcare.ahrq.gov /products/asthma-education/technical-brief

Allergy and Asthma Network. "Asthma and Exercise." https://allergy asthmanetwork.org/what-is-asthma/asthma-exercise/

Centers for Disease Control and Prevention. "Asthma Surveillance Data." https://www.cdc.gov/asthma/asthmadata.htm

Institute of Medicine. "Clearing the Air: Asthma and Indoor Air Exposure." https://pubmed.ncbi.nlm.nih.gov/25077220/

Organizations

Allergy and Asthma Network (AAN)

This national nonprofit network of families offers information about living with allergies and asthma. The website can help with your questions, concerns, and fears about asthma.

Website: https://allergyasthmanetwork.org/

Alliance of Community Health Plan (ACHP)

This organization works with medical directors, quality improvement staff, and other health plan officials to improve the health-care system and the lives of people in the communities they serve. The site provides background information about the intervention called "Asthma Intervention for Inner-City Children."

Website: https://achp.org/

Allies Against Asthma

Allies Against Asthma, a program of the Robert Woods Johnson Foundation, was a national initiative to improve asthma control for children and adolescents. This site provides tools and resources that may be useful to other asthma coalitions and programs addressing asthma.

Website: https://asthma.umich.edu/

American Academy of Allergy, Asthma, and Immunology (AAAAI)

If you think your child might have asthma, the first step is talking to a doctor or other medical professional. This website offers information about childhood asthma in English and Spanish.

Website: https://www.aaaai.org

American Academy of Family Physicians (AAFP)

This site provides information about asthma management and how to manage symptoms with an asthma action plan.

Website: https://www.aafp.or

American Academy of Pediatrics (AAP)

Asthma and allergies are among the most common chronic childhood diseases. It is important for family members to learn how to identify and avoid asthma and allergen triggers, recognize and present asthma attacks, understand medications, and help manage symptoms. This site offers information to help you learn more about childhood asthma and allergies.

Website: https://healthychildren.org

American Lung Association (ALA)

This organization works to improve lung health and prevent lung disease through Education, Advocacy and Research.

Website: https://lung.org

Asthma and Allergy Foundation of America

This nonprofit organization is dedicated to improving the quality of life for people with asthma and allergies and their caregivers. The site offers a multimedia library, a glossary of asthma terms, and a list of health professional programs educating and caring for patients with asthma.

Website: https://aafa.org

National Asthma Education and Prevention Program (NAEPP)

The National Asthma Education and Prevention Program works with other groups, including major medical associations, volunteer health organizations, and community programs, to educate patients, health professionals, and the public. This site contains information about the program, educational resources, and the *Expert Panel Report 3 (EPR3): Guidelines for the Diagnosis and Management of Asthma.*

Website: https://nhlbi.nih/science/national-asthma-education-and-prevent
ion.program

National Heart, Lung, and Blood Institute (NHLB)

This institute of the National Institutes of Health provides information for professionals and lay people on asthma.

Website: https: www.nhlbinih.gov/health-topics/asthma

National Institute of Allergy & Infectious Diseases (NIAID)

This site provides support for scientists conducting research aimed at developing better ways to diagnose, treat, and prevent asthma.

Website: https://www.niaid.nih.gov/

National Institute of Environmental Health Sciences (NIEHS)

This institute coordinates and supports research on environmental health sciences and provides resources.

Website: https://www.niehs.nih.gov/health/topics/conditions/asthma

National Jewish Medical and Research Center

This research center in Denver, Colorado, focuses on lung disorders, especially asthma.

Website: https://www.njc.org

National Library of Medicine (NLM)

The National Library of Medicine, the largest online medical library, provides health information, library services, research programs, and general information related to topics such as asthma.

Website: https://nlm.gov

U.S. Environmental Protection Agency (EPA)—Asthma Page

The EPA informs people about the environment and develops and enforces regulations about the environment. Its mission is to protect human health and the environment. Visit this website to learn about EPA's asthma education campaigns to promote asthma awareness in your community and the EPA National Environmental Leadership Awards.

Website: https://www.epa.gov/asthma

Bibliography

Abecasis, G. R., A. Auton, L. D. Brooks, et al. (2012). 1000 Genomes Project Consortium. An integrated map of genetic variation from 1,092 human genomes. *Nature* 491: 56–65.

Adams, F. (1849). *The Genuine Works of Hippocrates*. London: The Sydenham Society.

Aiello, A. E., R. M. Coulborn, V. Perez, and E. L. Larson. (2008). Effect of hand hygiene on infectious disease risk in the community setting: A meta-analysis. *Am J Public Health* 98(8): 1372–81.

Alwarith, J., H. Kahleova, L. Crosby, et al. (2020, March 13). The role of nutrition in asthma prevention and treatment. *Nutr Rev*: nuaa005. https://doi.org/10.1093/nutrit/nuaa005.

Amelink, M., S. Hashimoto, P. Spinhoven, et al. (2014, March). Anxiety, depression and personality traits in severe, prednisone-dependent asthma. *Respir Med* 108(3): 438–44.

American Asthma Foundation. (2020). The impact of asthma on society. https://www.americanasthmafoundation.org/impact-asthma.

Asthma Capitals. https://www.aafa.org/asthma-capitals. Accessed September 16, 2020.

Asthma in America 2018. (2020). What people fear most about their asthma. *Health Union*. https://health-union.com/blog/people-fear-future-asthma.

Atsjournals.org. (2018). The economic burden of asthma in the United States, 2008–2013. *Ann Am Thorac Soc*.https://www.atsjournals.org/doi/abs/10.1513/AnnalsATS.201703-259OC.

Bazhora, Y. I. (2020). Application of cognitive-behavioral therapy in patients with uncontrolled bronchial asthma due to excess body weight and obesity. *Wiad Lek* 73(1): 134–38.

Belanger, K., and E. W. Triche. (2008, August). Indoor combustion and asthma. *Immunol Allergy Clin North Am* 28(3): vii, 507–19. https://doi.org/10.1016/j.iac.2008.03.011.

Bell, J. T., and R. Saffery. (2012). The value of twins in epigenetic epidemiology. *Int J Epidemiol* 41: 140–50.

Bergstrom, J., S. M. Kurth, E. Bruhl, et al. Health care guideline: Diagnosis and management of asthma. 11th ed. *Institute for Clinical Systems Improvement.* www.icsi.org/wp-content/uploads/2019/01/Asthma.pdf. Updated December 2016. Accessed February 28, 2018.

Bisgaard, H., S. M. Jensen, and K. Bønnelykke. (2012). Interaction between asthma and lung function growth in early life. *Am J Respir Crit Care Med* 185: 1183–89.

Braman, S. S. (2006). The global burden of asthma. *Chest* 130(1 Suppl): 4–12.

Brazil, K., and P. Krueger. (2002). Patterns of family adaptation to childhood asthma. *J Pediatr Nurs* 17(3): 167–73.

Bronchial Thermoplasty. *Cleveland Clinic.* https://my.clevelandclinic.org/health/diseases/16811-bronchial-thermoplasty. Accessed November 2, 2020.

Calışkan, M., Y. A. Bochkov, E. Kreiner-Møller, et al. (2013). Rhinovirus wheezing illness and genetic risk of childhood-onset asthma. *N Engl J Med* 368: 1398–1407.

CDC.gov. (2018). CDC—Asthma—Data: Statistics, and surveillance. http://www.cdc.gov/asthma/asthmadata.htm.

Centers for Disease Control and Prevention. (2013, May 8). *National Vital Statistics Reports,* 61(4). https://www.cdc.gov/nchs/nvss/index.htm.

Centers for Disease Control and Prevention. (2015). Work-related asthma in 22 states. *MMWR Morb Mortal Wkly Rep* 64(13): 343.

Centers for Disease Control and Prevention. (2019). Asthma. *CDC.* https://www.cdc.gov/asthma/default.htm.

Chanez, P., and M. Humbert, eds. (2011). *L'Asthme Difficile: Questions Pratiques.* [Difficult Asthma: Practical Questions.] Paris: Phase 5.

Chang, T. S., R. F. Lemanske, T. W. Guilbert, et al. (2013). Evaluation of the modified asthma predictive index in high-risk preschool children. *J Allergy Clin Immunol Pract* 1: 152–56.

Charriot, J., I. Vachier, L. Halimi, et al. (2016). Future treatment for asthma. *Eur Respir Rev* 25: 77–92. https://doi.org/10.1183/16000617.0069-2015.

Clendenning, L. (1942). *Source Book of Medical History.* New York: Dover Publications.

Coffey, M. J., G. Sanders, W. L. Eschenbacher, et al. (1994). The role of methotrexate in the management of steroid-dependent asthma. *Chest* 105: 117–21.

Cookson, W. O. C. M., P. A. Sharp, J. A. Faux, and J. M. Hopkin. (1989). Linkage between immunoglobulin E responses underlying asthma and rhinitis and chromosome 11q. *Lancet* 333(8650): 1292–95.

Cukic, V., V. Lovre, and D. Dragisic. (2011). Sleep disorders in patients with bronchial asthma. *Mater Sociomed* 23(4): 235–37. https://doi.org /10.5455/msm.2011.23.235-237.

Dahl, R. (2006). Systemic side effects of inhaled corticosteroids in patients with asthma. *Respir Med* 100: 1307–17.

Dixon, A. E., and M. E. Poynter. (2016, May). Mechanisms of asthma in obesity: Pleiotropic aspects of obesity produce distinct asthma phenotypes. *Am J Respir Cell Mol Biol* 54(5): 601–8. https://doi.org.10 .1165/rcmb.2016-0017PS.

Dombret, M.-C., K. Alagha, and L. P. Boulet. (2014). Bronchial thermoplasty: A new therapeutic option for the treatment of severe, uncontrolled asthma in adults. *Eur Respir Rev* 23: 510–18.

Duijts, Liesbeth. (2012, January). Fetal and infant origins of asthma. *Eur J Epidemiol* 27(1): 5–14. Published online February 18, 2012. https:// doi.org/10.1007/s10654-012-9657-y.

Edris, A., S. De Feyter, and T. Maes, et al. (2019). Monoclonal antibodies in type 2 asthma: A systematic review and network meta-analysis. *Respir Res* 20: 179. https://doi.org/10.1186/s12931-019-1138-3.

Ernst, D. AirDuo Digihaler, a digital maintenance asthma inhaler therapy, gets FDA approval. airduodigihaler.com. Accessed November 9, 2020.

Etzel, R. (2003). How environmental exposures influence the development and exacerbation of asthma. *Pediatrics* 112(1 Pt 2): 233–9.

Gauvreau, G. M., L.-P. Boulet, R. Leigh, et al. (2015). A non-steroidal glucocorticoid receptor agonist inhibits allergen-induced late asthmatic responses. *Am J Respir Crit Care Med* 191: 161–67.

Gauvreau, G. M., J. M. Harris, L.-P. Boulet, et al. (2014). Targeting membrane-expressed IgE B cell receptor with an antibody to the M1 prime epitope reduces IgE production. *Sci Transl Med* 6: 243ra85.

Global Asthma Report 2018. A 88-page report on state-of-the-art treatment. www.globalasthmareport.org/. Accessed July 8, 2021.

Global Initiative for Asthma (GINA). *Global strategy for asthma management and prevention.* Update 2014 and Online Appendix. http:// www.ginasthma.org. Accessed November 12, 2019.

Gong, H. J. R. Famous allergy sufferer: Charles Dickens. *Achoo Allergy Blog.* https://www.achooallergy.com/learning/famous-asthma-sufferer. Accessed August 11, 2019.

Graft, D. F., and M. D. Valentine. (1993). Immunotherapy. In E. B. Weiss and M. Stein, eds., *Bronchial Asthma: Mechanisms and Therapeutics.* Boston: Little, Brown and Company, 934.

Grainge, C. L., L. C. K. Lau, J. A. Ward, et al. (2011). Effect of bronchoconstriction on airway remodeling in asthma. *N Engl J Med* 364:
2006–2015.

Grant, I. W. B. (1983). Asthma in New Zealand. *Br Med J* 286: 374–77.

Gray, C. L. (2020, January 16). Current controversies and future prospects
for peanut allergy prevention, diagnosis and therapies. *Dove Press*
2020: 51–66. https://doi.org/10.2147/JAA.S196268.

Halimi, L., P. Chanez, and M. Humbert. (2011). Quand l'asthme est difficile: C'est l'asthmatique qui a des difficultés psychologiques? [When
asthma is difficult: Is the asthmatic having psychological difficulties?] In P. Chanez and M. Humbert, eds., *L'Asthme Difficile: Questions Pratiques*. [Difficult Asthma: Practical Questions.] Paris:
Phase 5.

Hankin, C. S., A. Bronstone, Z. Wang, et al. (2013). Estimated prevalence
and economic burden of severe, uncontrolled asthma in the United
States. *J Allergy Clin Immunol* 131: AB126–AB100.

Herbarth, O., A. Marquis, A. Marquis, et al. (2015). Vaccination prevents
allergic disorders in children. *World Allergy Organ J* 8(Suppl 1):
A19. Published online April 8, 2015. https://doi.org/10.1186
/1939-4551-8-S1-A19.

Holgate, S. T., and A. M. Edwards. (2003). The chromones: Cromolyn
sodium and nedocromil sodium. In N. F. Adkinson, J. W. Yungin-
ger, W. W. Busse, et al., eds., *Middleton's Allergy: Principles and
Practice*, 6th ed. Mosby, St. Louis, 915.

Humbert, M., W. Busse, and N. A. Hanania. (2017, October). Controversies
and opportunities in severe asthma. *Curr Opin Pulm Med* 24(1): 1.
https://doi.org/10.1097/MCP.0000000000000438.

Interview with Jackie Joiner Kersee. (2011, Fall). *NIH Medline Plus*. https://
magazine.medlineplus.gov/pdf/MLP_Fall_11.pdf.

IOM (Committee on the Assessment of Asthma and Indoor Air of the
Institute of Medicine). (2000). *Clearing the Air: Asthma and Indoor
Air Exposures*. Washington, DC: National Academies Press. https://
download.nap.edu/login.php?record_id=9610&page=http%3A%2F
%2Fwww.nap.edu%2Fdownload.php%3Frecord_id%3D9610.

Irani, F., J. M. Barbone, J. Beausoleil, and L. Gerald. (2017). Is asthma associated with cognitive impairments. *J Clin Exp Neuropsychol*. https://
www.ncbi.nlm.nih.gov/m/pubmed/28325118/#.

Jutel, M., I. Agache, S. Bonini, et al. (2015). International consensus on
allergy immunotherapy. *J Allergy Clin Immunol* 136: 556–68.

Kabesch, M., S. Michel, and J. Tost. (2010). Epigenetic mechanisms and the
relationship to childhood asthma. *Eur Respir J* 36: 950–61.

Kallenbach, S., C. Babinet, S. Pournin, P. Cavelier, M. Goodhardt, and F.
Rougeon. (1993). The intronic immunoglobulin ϰ gene enhancer

acts independently on rearrangement and on transcription *Eur J Immunol* 23(8): 1917–21.

Kavuru, M., L. Pien, D. Litwin, S. Erzzurum, and M. Ahmad. (1995, September/October). Asthma: Current controversies and emerging therapies. *Clevel Clin J Med* 62(5): 293–304.

Kelkar, P. *Emotional and social effects of asthma.* https://blog.healthalliance .org/wellness-101/disease-management/emotional-and-social -effects-of-asthma/. Accessed August 18, 2020.

Kewalramani, A., M. E. Bollinger, and T. T. Postolache. (2008). Asthma and mood disorders. *Int J Child Health Hum Dev* 1(2): 115–23.

Kheirabadi, G., A. Malekian, and M. Fakharzadeh. (2007). Comparative study on the prevalence of depression in mothers with asthmatic, type I diabetic and healthy children. *J Res Behav Sci* 5(1): 21–25. (Persian.)

Kieckhefer, G. M., and M. Ratcliffe. (2000). What parents of children with asthma tell us. *J Pediatr Health Care* 14(3): 122–26.

Klein, M., A. Magnan, and G. Bouchaud. (2019, April). Allergen-derived peptide: A promising approach in asthma. *Rev Mal Respir* 36(4): 442–46. https://doi.org/10.1016/j.rmr.2019.03.005. Epub April 18, 2019. (Abstract in English, article in French.)

Knarborg, M., Ole H., H.-J. Hoffmann, and Ronald Dahl. (2014). Methotrexate as an oral corticosteroid-sparing agent in severe asthma: The emergence of a responder asthma endotype. *Eur Clin Respir J* 1: 10.3402/ecrj.v1.25037. Published online November 14, 2014. https:// doi.org/10.3402/ecrj.v1.25037.

Kulalert, P., P. Phinyo, J. Patumanond, et al. (2020). Continuous versus intermittent short-acting β2-agonists nebulization as first-line therapy in hospitalized children with severe asthma exacerbation: A propensity score matching analysis. *Asthma Res Pract* 6: 6. Published online July 2, 2020. https://doi.org/10.1186/s40733-020-00059-5.

Lavorini, F., C. Janson, F. Braido, G. Stratelis, and A. Løkke. (2019, January–December). What to consider before prescribing inhaled medications: A pragmatic approach for evaluating the current inhaler landscape. *Ther Adv Respir Dis* 13:1753466619884532. https://doi .org/10.1177/1753466619884532. PMID: 31805823; PMCID: PMC 6900625.

Leaker, B. R., D. Singh, S. Lindgren, et al. (2019). Effects of the toll-like receptor 7 (TLR7) agonist, AZD8848, on allergen-induced responses in patients with mild asthma: A double-blind, randomised, parallel-group study. *Respir Res* 20: 288. https://doi.org/10.1186/s12931-019 -1252-2.

Lindgren, S., L. Belin, S. Dreborg, E. Eisarsson, and I Pahlman. (1988). *Breed-specific dog-dandruff allergens. EPA Links between outdoor air pollution and childhood asthma.* https://www.epa.gov/sciencematters /links-between-air-pollution-and-childhood-asthma.

Littenberg, B. (1988). Aminophylline treatment in severe, acute asthma: A meta-analysis. *JAMA* 259: 1678–84.

Mapp, C. E., P. Boschetto, P. Maestrelli, and L. M. Fabbri. (2005, August 1). Occupational asthma. *Am J Respir Crit Care Med* 172(3): 280–305. https://doi.org/10.1164/rccm.200311-1575SO. Epub April 28, 2005.

Marin, G., A. S. Gamez, N. Molinari, et al. (2013). Distal airway impairment in obese normoreactive women. *BioMed Res Int* 2013: 707856.

Mayo Clinic. https://www.mayoclinic.org/diseases-conditions/asthma/in -depth/asthma-inhalers/art-20046382. Accessed January 30, 2020.

McFadden, E. R. (2004, August). A century of asthma. *Am J Respir Crit Care Med* 170(3): 251–21.

Merz, E.-M., N. S. Consedine, H.-J. Schulze, and C. Schuengel. (2009). Well-being of adult children and ageing parents: Associations with intergenerational support and relationship quality. *Ageing & Society* 29: 783–802. https://doi.org/10.1017/s0144686x09008514.

Microbiology Society Press release. (2019, March 28). *The hygiene hypothesis is out of date and is undermining public health.* https:// microbiologysociety.org /news /press -releases /the -hygiene -hypothesis-is-out-of-date-and-is-undermining-public-health.html.

Mirershadi, F., M. Ahmadi, A. Rezabakhsh, et al. (2020). Unraveling the therapeutic effects of mesenchymal stem cells in asthma. *Stem Cell Res Ther* 11: 400. https://doi.org/10.1186/s13287-020-01921-2.

Mitchell, D. K. (2015). *Asthma and school functioning in children: Still work to do.* https://onlinelibrary.wiley.com/doi/abs/10.1002/cbl .30064.

Mitchell, D., and K. K. Murdock. (2002). Self-competence and coping in urban children with asthma. *Child Health Care* 31(4): 273–93.

Moffatt, M. F., I. G. Gut, F. Demenais, et al. (2010). A large-scale, consortium-based genomewide association study of asthma. *N Engl J Med* 363: 1211.

Murphy, L. K., C. B. Murray, and B. E. Compas; ed. C. A. Gerhardt, C. A. Berg, D. J. Wiebe, and G. N. Holmbeck. (2017, January 1). Topical review: Integrating findings on direct observation of family communication in studies comparing pediatric chronic illness and typically developing samples. *J Pediatr Psychol* 42(1): 85–94. https://doi .org/10.1093/jpepsy/jsw051. PMID: 28172942.

National Heart, Lung, and Blood Institute. (2007). Guidelines for the diagnosis and treatment of asthma. Expert panel 3 report. https:// getasthmahelp.org/documents/Trifold_EssentialInformation _85x11Finalrev.pdf.

National Heart, Lung, and Blood Institute, National Asthma Education Program. (1991). Expert panel report. Guidelines for the diagnosis and management of asthma. *Allerg Chin Immunol* 88: 425–534.

Nunes, C., A. M. Pereira, and M. Morais-Almeida. (2017). Asthma costs and social impact. *Asthma Res Pract* 3(1). https://doi.org/10.1186 /s40733-016-0029-3.

Nwaru, B. I., M. Ekström, P. Hasvold, et al. (2020). Overuse of short-acting β2-agonists in asthma is associated with increased risk of exacerbation and mortality: A nationwide cohort study of the global SABINA programme. *Eur Respir J* 55: 1901872. https://doi.org/10 .1183/13993003.01872-2019.

Okada, H., C. Kuhn, H. Feillet, and J.-F. Bach. (2010, April). The "hygiene hypothesis" for autoimmune and allergic diseases: An update. *Clin Exp Immunol* 160(1): 1–9. https://doi.org/10.1111/j.1365-2249.2010 .04139.x.

Phulke, S., S. Kaushik, S. Kaur, and S. S. Pandav. (2017). Steroid-induced glaucoma: An avoidable irreversible blindness. *J Curr Glaucoma Pract* 11(2): 67–72.

Platts-Mills, T., J. Vaughan, S. Squillace, J. Woodfolk, and R. Sporik. (2001). Sensitisation, asthma, and a modified Th2 response in children exposed to cat allergen: A population-based cross-sectional study. *Lancet* 357(9258): 752–6.

Pleskovic, N., A. Bartholow, D. A. Gentile, and D. P. Skoner. (2015, August). The future of sublingual immunotherapy in the United States. *Curr Allergy Asthma Rep* 15(8): 44. https://doi.org/10.1007/s11882-015 -0545-x.

Poitiers University Hospital. (2015). *Evaluation of a therapeutic strategy including nebulised liposomal amphotericin B (Ambisome®) in maintenance treatment of allergic bronchopulmonary aspergillosis (cystic fibrosis excluded).* (NEBULAMB). https://clinicaltrials.gov /ct2/show/NCT02273661.

Porpodis, K., P. Zarogoulidis, D. Spyratos, et al. (2014, March). Pneumothorax and asthma. *J Thorac Dis* 6(Suppl 1): S152–S161. https://soi .org/10.3978/j.issn.2072-1439.2014.03.05.

Porter, Roy. (1997a). *The Greatest Benefit to Mankind: A Medical History of Humanity.* New York: W. W. Norton.

Porter, Roy. (1997b). *Medicine: A History of Healing.* New York: Barnes and Noble Books.

Rees, J. (2005). Methods of delivering drugs. *BMJ* 331(7515): 504–6. https:// doi.org/10.1136/bmj.331.7515.504.

Robertson, C. F. (2002, September 16). Long-term outcome of childhood asthma. *Med J Aust* 177(S6): S42–S44.

Sakula, Alex. (1988, January). A history of asthma. *J R Coll Physicians Lond* 22(1): 36–44.

Sandford, A. J., and P. D. Pare. (2000). The genetics of asthma: The important questions. *ATS J.* https://doi.org/10.1164/ajrccm.161.supplement_2.a1q4-11.

Schuijs, M. J., M. A. Willart, K. Vergote, et al. (2015). Farm dust and endotoxin protect against allergy through A20 induction in lung epithelial cells. *Science* 349: 1106–10.

Scudellari, M. (2017, February 14). News feature: Cleaning up the hygiene hypothesis. *PNAS* 114(7): 1433–36. https://doi.org/10.1073/pnas.1700688114.

Shusterman, Dennis. (1992). *Health effects of environmental odor pollution.* https://www.researchgate.net/profile/Dennis_Shusterman/publication/21615734_Critical_Review_The_Health_Significance_of_Environmental_Odor_Pollution/links/53e66ea00cf21cc29fd4d6bb.pdf.

Slager, R. E., G. A. Hawkins, E. J. Ampleford, et al. (2010). IL-4 receptor α polymorphisms are predictors of a pharmacogenetic response to a novel IL-4/IL-13 antagonist. *J Allergy Clin Immunol* 126: 875–78.

Spitzer, W. O., S. Suissa, P. Ernest, et al. (1992). The use of B-agonists and the risk of death and near death from asthma. *N Engl J Med* 326: 501–06.

Stephenson, Laurel. (2017, November). Monoclonal antibody therapy for asthma. *Clin Pulm Med* 24(6): 250–57. https://doi.org/10.1097/CPM.0000000000000234.

Strachan, D. P. (1989). Hay fever, hygiene, and household size. *BMJ* 299: 1259–60.

Sur, S., T. B. Crotty, G. M. Kephart, et al. (1993). Sudden-onset fatal asthma. *Am Rev Respir Dis* 148: 713–19.

Świerczyńska-Krępa, M., M. Sanak, G. Bochenek, et al. (2014). Aspirin desensitization in patients with aspirin-induced and aspirin-tolerant asthma: A double-blind study. *J Allergy Clin Immunol* 134: 883–90.

Thomas, M., and C. Griffiths. *Asthma and panic scope for intervention?* https://www.atsjournals.org/doi/full/10.1164/rccm.2503005 Accessed November 19, 2002.

Thomas, P. A., H. Liu, and D. Umberson. (2017, November). Family relationships and well-being. *Innov Aging* 1(3): igx025. Published online November 11, 2017. https://doi.org/10.1093/geroni/igx025.

Thomsen, S. (2015a). The contribution of twin studies to the understanding of the aetiology of asthma and atopic diseases. *Eur Clin Respir J* 2: 10.3402/ecrj.v2.27803. Published online September 11, 2015. https://doi.org/10.3402/ecrj.v2.27803.

Thomsen, S. (2015b). Genetics of asthma: An introduction for the clinician. *Eur Clin Respir J* 2: 10.3402/ecrj.v2.24643. Published online January 16, 2015. https://doi.org/10.3402/ecrj.v2.24643.

Tursynbek, A. N., and J. A. Krishnan. (2019, November). What will uncontrolled asthma cost in the United States? *Am J Respir Crit Care Med* 200(9): 1077–78.

2020 Focused Update to the Asthma Management Guidelines. https://www.nhlbi.nih.gov/sites/default/files/media/docs/NAEPPCC Guidelines Update. Accessed November 9, 2020.

U.S. Food and Drug Administration. Asthma: The hygiene hypothesis. Content current as of March 23, 2018. https://www.fda.gov/vaccines -blood-biologics/consumers-biologics/asthma-hygiene-hypothesis.

Wahls, S. A. (2012). Causes and evaluation of chronic dyspnea. *Am Fam Phys* 86: 173–82. http://www.aafp.org/afp/2012/0715/p173.pdf.

Wang, L., M. Feng, Q. Li, C. Qiu, and R. Chen. (2019, April). Advances in nanotechnology and asthma. *Ann Transl Med* 7(8): 180. https://doi .org/10.21037/atm.2019.04.62.

Wang, Y., J. Chen, W. Chen, et al. (2021). Does asthma increase the mortality of patients with COVID-19?: A systematic review and meta-analysis. *Int Arch Allergy Immunol.* https://doi.org/10.1159/000510953.

Warrington, R. (2010). Immunotherapy in asthma. *Immunotherapy* 2(5): 711–25.

Wasserfallen, J. B., M. D. Schaller, F. Feihl, et al. (1995). Sudden asphyxic asthma: A distinct entity? *Am Rev Respir Dis* 14(2): 108–11.

Wechsler, M. E. (2006). Managing asthma in the 21st century: Role of pharmacogenetics. *Pediatr Ann* 35:660–62, 664–69.

What is associated with pediatric mortality? *Medscape.* https://www .medscape.com/answers/1000997-78372/what-is-the-mortality -and-morbidity-associated-with-pediatric-asthma. Accessed January 31, 2020.

Wood, R. A., P. A. Eggleston, P. Lind, et al. (1988). Antigenic analysis of household dust samples. *Am Rev Respir Dis* 137: 358.

Wood, R. A., A. N. Laheri, and P. A. Eggleston. (1993, September). The aerodynamic characteristics of cat allergen. *Clin Exp Allergy* 23(9): 733–39.

Wright, R. J., M. Rodriguez, and S. Cohen. (1998). Review of psychosocial stress and asthma: An integrated biopsychosocial approach. *Thorax* 53:1066–74. https://www.ncbi.nlm.nih.gov/pmc/articles/PMC1745142/pdf/v053 p01066.pdf.

Yale Center for Asthma and Airway Disease. (2020). *Bronchial thermoplasty.* https://medicine.yale.edu/intmed/pulmonary/ycaad/clinical _center/bronchial-thermoplasty/.

Yorke, J., P. Adair, A.-M. Doyle, et al. (2017, June). A randomised controlled feasibility trial of group cognitive behavioural therapy for people with severe asthma. *J Asthma* 54(5): 543–54. https://doi.org/10.1080/02770903.2016.1229335.

Yuksel, H., A. Sogut, O. Yilmaz, et al. (2012). Role of adipokines and hormones of obesity in childhood asthma. *Allergy Asthma Immunol Res* 4: 98–103.

Zein, J., and S. C. Erzurum. (2015, June). Asthma is different in women. *Curr Allergy Asthma Rep* 15(6): 28. https://doi.org/10.1007/s11882-015-0528-y.

Zhernov, Y., M. Curin, M. Khaitov, A. Karaulov, and R. Valenta. (2019, August). Recombinant allergens for immunotherapy: State of the art. *Curr Opin Allergy Clin Immunol* 19(4): 402–14. https://doi.org/10.1097/ACI.0000000000000536.

Index

About the Author

Evelyn B. Kelly, PhD, is a medical writer, speaker, and educator. She has a PhD from the University of Florida, Gainesville; a master's degree in religion from the Southern Baptist Theological Seminary; and a bachelor's degree in English and microbiology from the University of Tennessee. However, her favorite subjects are history, travel, and political science.

She has written over 400 articles, and this volume on asthma is her 20th book. Her recent books for ABC-CLIO include *Stem Cells, Obesity, Encyclopedia of Attention Deficit Hyperactivity Disorders, The 101 Most Unusual Diseases and Disorders*, the two-volume *Encyclopedia of Human Genetics and Disease, Gene Therapy*, and *The Skeletal System*. Evelyn lives on a farm in Ocala, Florida. She has four children, four grandchildren, and four great-grandchildren. She has traveled to 85 countries and has visited all seven continents.